Fundamental Aspects of Mental Health Nursing

Edited by
James Dooher

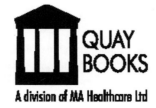

QUAY
BOOKS

A division of MA Healthcare Ltd

Quay Books Division, MA Healthcare Ltd, St Jude's Church, Dulwich Road, London
SE24 0PB

British Library Cataloguing-in-Publication Data
A catalogue record is available for this book

© MA Healthcare Limited 2008
ISBN-10: 1 85642 197 X; ISBN-13: 978 1 85642 197 3

Printed by Athenaeum Press Ltd, Dukes Way, Team Valley, Gateshead, NE11 OPZ

Contents

Contributors

James Alexander, Clinical Manager, Nottingham Healthcare NHS Trust

Oduth Chooramun, Senior Lecturer, Faculty of Health and Life Sciences, De Montfort University, Leicester

Jacqui Day is Senior Lecturer at De Montfort University, Leicester

James Dooher, Principal Lecturer and Academic Lead for Mental Health Nursing, De Montfort University, Leicester

Kelvin Ford, Senior Lecturer in Mental Health, Psychology and Sociology of Health, De Montfort University, Leicester

Dave Kingdon, Senior Practice Therapist, Common Mental Health Problem Service, Leicestershire

Daniel Kinnair, Specialist Registrar in General Adult Psychiatry, Leicestershire Partnership NHS Trust, and Visiting Lecturer, De Montfort University, Leicester

Barbara Monk-Steel, Senior Lecturer in Mental Health Nursing, De Montfort University, Leicester

Godfrey Moyo, Senior Lecturer in Mental health Nursing, De Montfort University, Leicester

Paul Rigby, Senior Lecturer in Nursing at De Montfort University, Leicester. He is also a Community Mental Health Nurse, Leicestershire Partnership NHS Trust

Sally Rudge, Chartered Counselling Psychologist, Derby Hospitals NHS Foundation Trust

John Unsworth-Webb, Consultant in Health Care Education, London

This book is dedicated to Albert Goddard,
an unsung hero of the service user movement

Introduction

Mental health nurses care for people with mental health problems in the community or sometimes in a hospital setting. They help patients lead as 'normal' a life as possible, striving to enable the optimum potential of those they work with. /

The mindset of mental health nursing has shifted from that of a psychiatric nurse, whose primary function was to carry out 'doctors orders' and deliver the prescribed treatment to the patient, towards an evidence-based, health orientated leader of care, practicing in a diverse range of settings.

This book sets out to provide the reader with an insight into some of the fundamental elements of good quality mental health nursing in an accessible format. The themes will cover some of the physical, psychological, social and spiritual elements of quality mental health, and the part nurses play in their promotion.

Mental health nursing, sometimes referred to as psychiatric nursing, is a branch of the nursing profession that cares for people of all ages suffering from mental distress. Mental health nurses occupy the largest proportion of any other profession working in mental health services today (CNO, 2006), and utilize a wide range of skills, therapies and resources to help and support people in their daily lives. Assisting people resolve their own problems is a fundamental part of mental health nursing, and the types of problem people suffer from vary enormously. Mental health nurses make a vital contribution to providing care to service users of all age groups and in all settings.

The prevalence and frequency of mental health problems in the UK is statistically well documented, although as with all statistics they should be treated with caution. Depending on the research organisation, some figures suggest that it could be expected that 1 in 6 people will suffer some form of mental distress during their lifetime (Singleton et al, 2000). Traditionally, this distress may require the help of a professional if it becomes severe or threatens the safety of the person or other people, however, most mental health problems do not fall into this category.

Contemporary services aim to provide support that is easily accessible and meets the individual's needs. This localised service revolves around the GP surgery in what is described as Primary Care, or where absolutely necessary within a hospital setting.

The developments leading to this community focus for care were prompted by the closure of the institutions in the late 1980s. This saw in a new era for mental health nursing and a change of focus from providing continuing and long-term care in places removed from mainstream society, into more home based patient centred care.

The development of self-help, complementary medicine and computer-based therapy, has been reflected positively through the populations' increased understanding and empowered status. The progress towards informed decisions, however, is hampered by the range and choice of service offered by private, public and voluntary sectors. Although the incidence of poor mental health cuts across social divides, it is particularly evident for those described as 'socially excluded'. Their failure to engage voluntarily with the system does not suggest being overwhelmed by choice, rather it may reflect the difficultly they have in accessing services.

For some people the choice of receiving services is removed if they are detained under the Mental Health Act. About 1% of the population experience a disorder of perception (often referred to as schizophrenia at some point in their lives (Mental Health Foundation, 1999), and about 1% of the population experience manic depression at some point in their lives (Mental Health Foundation, 1999). Singleton et al (2000) suggested that 1 in 200 people have experienced a psychotic illness in the last year. For many people the experience of symptoms traditionally associated with mental illness will be a single event, and this does not necessarily indicate the need for a diagnosis. A first episode may well relate to a range of contributory external factors which if addressed will promote a complete and permanent recovery.

Recurrent symptoms may indicate the need for engagement with mental health services, and it is with this population that the majority of mental health nursing takes place.

In recent years mental health nursing has been shaped by a number of documents which feature in this book, but perhaps one of the most influential is the *National Service Framework for Mental Health* (DH, 1999a). It addresses the mental health needs of working age adults up to 65 and sets out national standards, national service models, local action, and national underpinning programmes for implementation. It is explicit that the majority of mental health problems are best dealt with in primary care, and presents Primary Care Trusts and primary care providers with some significant challenges:

- Providing primary care to the socially excluded, for example those with drug and mental health problems
- Development of professional skills and knowledge to deal effectively with mental health problems
- Providing information about available resources (social, welfare and voluntary resources)
- Addressing the physical healthcare needs of users

- Coordinating systems to enable communication between all stakeholders involved in the care of a user, leading to maximised outcomes for the individual with consistent advice
- Implementation of care pathways and protocols to enhance clinical outcomes
- Measurement of user experiences and performance against national target
- Meeting carers' needs
- Suicide risk management

Mental health nurses need to be prepared to play their part in these successful outcomes, and it is through education, training and collaboration with other disciplines that will determine the success of these aspirations.

Mental Health Nurse Education

To qualify as a mental health nurse, you need to complete a three-year university course which has been approved by the Nursing and Midwifery Council (NMC) and specialises in mental health. Most courses are equally split between theory (50%) and practice (50%).

Nursing diploma and degree courses are available within most universities in the UK. The degree and diploma pathways both provide the same amount of practical experience, but degree courses are perhaps more suited to those who enjoy the academic challenge of exploring the theoretical side of mental health nursing in greater depth. Additionally, some universities offer an NMC approved Advanced Diploma in Nursing. This qualification and the entry requirements for it lie between diploma and degree level.

All pre-registration nursing courses are based upon a set of recommendations and regulations as specified in: *Fitness for Practice* (NMC [formerly the UKCC], 1999), *Making a Difference* (DH, 1999), and documents such as the *National Service Framework for Mental Health* (DH 1999, 2004) and *Standards for Proficiency* (NMC, 2006). This set of benchmarks ensures the consistency in the quality of nurse training and education. This is supported by Wilshaw (2004), who proposed that mental health nurses now fulfill a wider range of responsibilities than ever before, that nursing is more important than ever, and that student nurses are — at least in principle — better prepared than ever.

There are no national minimum entry requirements because each university has its own criteria, however to get onto an approved course you need to meet some general requirements set by the NMC, which include:

- Providing evidence of your literacy and numeracy, good health and good character, and recent successful study experience
- Meeting the minimum age requirement for nurse training (17.5 years old in England, 17 in Scotland, and 18 in Northern Ireland and Wales)
- Agreeing to have a criminal records bureau check (a criminal conviction does not automatically exclude you from working within the NHS).

Previous education requirements are generally around five GCSEs or equivalent at grade C or above, including in English language or literature and a science subject for a Diploma programme, and five GCSEs and two A-levels or equivalent for a Degree programme.

Universities across the country have made great efforts to what they describe a 'widening the entry gate' to enable a person with potential who has not come by traditional educational routes has a fair chance of accessing the programme. Previous experience, paid or unpaid, of working with people who use mental health services will always be of benefit to the prospective applicant

Alternatives, such as an Access to Higher Education course, may be accepted by some institutions.Some universities offer a "Cadet" scheme for 16 to 19 years olds who can prepare for a career in nursing by doing a two-year Cadet Scheme. The scheme includes clinical placements and working towards a qualification such as an NVQ Level 3 in Health, or Health and Social Care.

Another entry route is enabled by working in a caring role, for example as a healthcare assistant or support worker, where the NHS Trust or employer may sponsor the person to gain the necessary entry requirements and in some cases second that person to undertake their nurse training by topping up the bursary to ensure that their previous salary is maintained.

Overseas trained nurses may need to complete the NMC approved Overseas Nurses Programme (ONP) in order to begin professional practice in the UK.

Generally, criteria can and do vary, and it is advisable that any applicant ensures they meet the requirements of the local area to which they apply.

The Diploma of Higher Education in Nursing and BSc(Hons) Nursing courses offered by universities are full-time three-year programmes that have a Common Foundation element in the first year, which gives students a taste and flavour of all branches of nursing and prepares them in terms of safe practice and professional expectations. These courses have some common aspirations, which can be briefly described as:

- To produce knowledgeable, professionally able students who are equipped to meet the changing needs of the health service

- To provide educational opportunities, which support careers in each of the nursing pathways
- To fulfil the statutory and professional requirements for pre-registration qualifications in nursing
- To provide opportunities to acquire a relevant knowledge base in nursing and appropriate practice skills
- To produce knowledgeable students, skilled in IT and use of health information, who are able to critique, and analyse theory related to nursing and nursing practice
- To facilitate the opportunity for students to utilise nursing theory and research in professional practice.

Practical work experience with patients is supported by a trained Mentor who is able to guide the student in becoming a safe and effective practitioner. Students need to demonstrate the capability and competence both in the classroom and in the practice setting, and every university has a set of criteria that the student must achieve to progress within the course and eventually register with the NMC.

Responsibilities of the Mental Health Nurse

Mental health nurses are at the front line in providing care and support in both hospitals and the community. Since the late 1980s there has been a significant shift from hospital to the community as the setting for mental health care. Nurses now work in people's homes, in small residential units, and in local health centres. Nurses work as part of a multidisciplinary team which incorporates psychiatrists, social workers, psychologists, GPs, occupational therapists and others to co-ordinate care.

At the heart of mental health nursing care is the one-to-one personal relationship that nurses develop with their patients. This is achieved through a combination of good communication skills, knowledge of the person and their presenting symptoms together with an ability to observe behaviour, and try to work out the underlying emotions and feelings (affect), and thinking (cognitions) that have produced that behaviour. There is a range of well documented range of activities that are associated with developing a therapeutic rapport and a plan of care interventions which meet that patient's specific needs. Typical work activities include:

- Listening to patients and interpreting their needs and concerns
- Assessing and talking to patients offering explanation and reassurance about treatment they are receiving

- Caring for patients who are acutely unwell or have a long standing or enduring mental health problem
- Building relationships with patients to encourage trust
- Ensuring the correct administration of medication, including injections, and monitoring the results of treatment
- Responding to distressed patients and attempting to understand the source of their distress in a non-threatening manner
- Advocating for a patient who may temporarily not be able to adequately represent their own best interests
- Participating in group and/or one-to-one therapy sessions, both as an individual and with other health professionals;
- Encouraging patients to take part in art, drama or occupational therapy where appropriate
- Organising social events aimed at developing patients' social skills
- Devising plans of care that anticipate risks, and promote the safety, health and well being of the patient
- Maintaining patient records and evaluating care plans
- Applying the 'de-escalation' approach to help people manage their emotions and behaviour
- Ensuring that the legal requirements appropriate to a particular setting or group of patients are observed.

As a mental health nurse you are likely to be dealing with people from a broad range of social, economic and cultural backgrounds, and the understanding of these factors is a critical element in building a therapeutic relationship. One difference between nurses and other mental health workers is that nurses are able to forge a long standing relationships, often spending much longer periods of time working with patients and thereby developing the trust essential to effective mental health care.

Ward and Community Work

Registered mental health nurses tend to work either in a community environment or ward environment. This simple division can be generally be identified as either Primary of Secondary Care. The Department of Health defines primary health care as all those health services provided outside hospital by family health services, and include the four practitioner services of GPs, dentists, community pharmacists and opticians. In addition, primary care incorporates community health services which include, midwives, health visitors and some nurses, chiropodists and physiotherapists.

Primary care services provide the medical care a patient receives upon first contact with the healthcare system, before referral elsewhere within the system. Conversely Secondary health care refers to specialist services that may be either community- or hospital-based but are reliant upon the screening and subsequent referral from one of their primary care colleagues.

Community Work

Community Mental Health Teams generally comprise of community mental health nurses, a psychiatrist, social workers, and community workers working in partnership with other disciplines, agencies and carers to provide home based services for clients and their families. Where possible, realistic alternatives to hospital are sought, and for those who have been admitted into hospital care, these teams work with the person to ease their discharge process and plan a package of care for when they return home.

Community Mental Health Teams mostly work with people between the ages of 18 to 65 with mental health difficulties. Their role may involve:

- Co-ordinating the care of patients
- Liaising with patients, relatives and fellow professionals in the community treatment team and attending regular meetings to review and monitor patients' care plans
- Visiting patients in their home to monitor progress
- Assessing patients' behaviour and psychological needs
- Identifying if and when a patient is at risk of harming themselves or others.

These activities support a range of general aims which set out to:

- Reduce the number of re-admissions to hospital by earlier intervention and identification of problems
- Reduce the number of people in hospital by having staff with the necessary skills working within the community
- Develop services which are responsive and support the person to reach their optimum potential in the home environment
- Work closely with the voluntary and independent services, ensuring that the appropriate interventions are offered
- Support a close working relationship between relevant professionals resulting in a quicker comprehensive assessment of needs and the package of care.

The generic nature of Community Mental Health Teams has led to some aspects of their role being devolved to specialist teams. The interventions involved in crisis work, for example, is often taken up by a crisis resolution service, whereas work with people in recovery is undertaken by Assertive Outreach Teams (Dooher, 2006). Older people have specialist teams too, and young peoples services are delivered by Child and Adolescent Mental Health Services (CAMHS).

Working in a Ward Environment

When working in a ward environment, the primary nurse (staff nurse) is generally responsible for the assessment of care needs using a nursing process (assessment planning implementation and evaluation) format to develop programmes of care for a small inpatient case load. The nurse will regularly take charge of the ward and provide supervision, mentorship and leadership for staff other staff a student nurses. Staff Nurses work closely with ward manager and senior staff in using evidence-based practice in delivery of care. Some of the key tasks and responsibilities include:

- Assessing individual care needs, developing care plans, delivering nursing care and evaluating outcomes
- Being an effective listener observer and communicator
- Maintaining patient confidentiality at all times
- Adhering to all organisational, policies, procedures and guidelines
- Ensuring good working relationships with patients, carers, relatives, other professionals and the public
- Demonstrating an understanding to the use of clinical supervision to reflect upon and modify practice
- Ensuring that practice remains within legal, ethical and professional parameters and is open to scrutiny from peers.

Clinically, ward-based staff nurses should respond to the needs of people in an honest, non-judgemental and open manner, which respects the rights of individuals and groups, whilst actively engaging with patients in the provision of holistic, needs-led care that takes account of the physical, psychological, emotional, social and spiritual needs of individuals and groups.

As with all nursing posts, the ward-based nurse should demonstrate a commitment to equal opportunities for all people, and understand the impact of social and cultural diversity on patients' and carers' experiences of mental illness and mental health services. They need to respond to the needs of people sensitively with regard to age, culture, race, gender, ethnicity, religion and disability, especially regarding patients' privacy and dignity. In addition, understanding the rights of patients and carers and assisting them in exercising those rights.

Undertaking daily care in support of a written plan of care, reporting on care delivery and documenting it is a key factor in the transmission of information between staff, demonstrating the ability to work collaboratively, and having good self-awareness. This will enhance the nurses' ability to develop therapeutic relationships, incorporating limit and boundary setting, and implementing evidence-based practice using a range of assessment and measuring tools and risk management.

Good observational skills, and good verbal and non-verbal communication skills, are part of the key skill set needed to facilitate patients' use of effective treatment through negotiation skills, provision of information, assessment, management and systematic monitoring of side effects.

Key Challenges

There are a number of key challenges that mental health nurse face. Barker (2005) suggests that, compared to the prominent positions adopted by psychiatric medicine, psychology, social work and even the voluntary sector groups like Mind or Rethink, mental health nursing is pitifully represented in the media if not absent altogether. He goes on to observe that mental health nursing is like a sleeping giant, awaiting some magical event to rouse it from its slumbers.

One of the main challenges to mental health nursing is the objective improving outcomes for service users (DH, 2006). In her review of the profession, the Chief Nursing Officer recommended that the development and sustenance of positive therapeutic relationships with service users, their families and/or carers should form the basis of all care.

Mental health needs to move away from a medical model where it is the diagnosis that dictates the treatment experience of the service user, and embrace what is described as a holistic approach. A holistic approach to health differs from the conventional medical approach in that it takes into account the whole patient rather than just focusing on the symptom or the part that has the problem, and recognizes that the emotional, psychological, spiritual, social, cultural and physical elements of each person comprise a system, and therefore attempts to treat the whole person in his or her context.

This means that mental health nurses need to develop their skill and knowledge set to provide evidence-based psychological therapies, better assessment and health promotion activities that form the basis of care plans to meet the complex demands of individual patients.

Mental health nursing may also be under threat from the development of inter-professional education (IPE). On the surface, IPE is a positive development and an uncritical assumption that occasions when two or more professions learn with, from and about each other, to improve collaboration, and the quality of care, is a positive thing. If we scratch the veneer beneath it, however, we can acknowledge the positives, but also see that the lust for greater IPE may be driven by economic issues (for example economies of scale dictate that it is cheaper to teach a group of 200 than a group of 35), and the gradual erosion of the mental health nurses role. IPE is now a firm part of mainstream education at the pre-qualifying stage for many students in the health and social care professions. Freeth et al (2005), and although the benefits of understanding each other's roles and responsibilities will improve patient care, there is an inevitability that the specialist elements of separate professional roles are being challenged. This is particularly evident when we overlay the proposed role changes and increased responsibilities for mental health nurses contained within the largely discredited Mental Health Bill. The natural development of IPE is that as we see it grow we se collaborative learning and experience pathways develop and the convergence of the roles and responsibilities for Social Workers, Occupational Therapists, doctors, psychologists and mental health nurses. The outcome may be a generic worker who is able to prescribe medicine, hold people against their will, nurse them and provide a range of psychological therapies.

Whilst it is acknowledged that mental health nurses have a skill base that is already multifaceted, these new additions will see a reduced need for multidisciplinary working because all the elements of the team will be contained within a single individual. If mental health nurses are to use their specialist skills and personal strengths to uphold the uniqueness of their profession and help people come to terms with their problems, then they must focus on the most important factor within their toolbox; the therapeutic relationship, the ability to listen and draw information out, helping people find means of coping with their problems, and coordinating a patient's care.

References

Barker P (2005) *It's time the giant of mental health nursing woke up.* Psychominded.co.uk. http://www.psychminded.co.uk/news/news (accessed 16 May 2006)

CNO (2006) *Values to Action: The Chief Nursing Officer's Review of Mental Health Nursing.* HMSO, London

Dooher J (2006) *New Ways of Working in Mental Health.* Quay Books, Dinton Salisbury

DH (1999) *Making a Difference: Strengthening the Nursing, Midwifery and Health Visiting Contribution to Health and Healthcare.* HMSO, London

DH (1999a) *National Service Framework for Mental Health.* HMSO, London

DH (2004) *National Service Framework for Mental Health: Five Years On.*

DH (2006) *From Values to Action: The Chief Nursing Officer's Review of Mental Health Nursing*. DH, London

Mental Health Foundation (1999) *Fundamental Facts*. Mental Health Foundation, London

NMC (2004) *NMC Code of Professional Conduct: Standards for Conduct, Performance and Ethics*. NMC, London

NMC (2006) *Standards to Support Learning and Assessment in Practice: NMC Standards for Mentors, Practice Teachers and Teachers*. NMC, London

Singleton N, Bumpstead R, O'Brien M, Lee A, Meltzer H (2000) *Psychiatric Morbidity Among Adults Living in Private Households, 2000: Summary Report*. Office for National Statistics, London

Wilshaw G (2004) *Consultant Nursing in Mental Health*. Kingsham, Chichester

UKCC (1999) *Fitness for Practice: The UKCC Commission for Nursing and Midwifery Education 1999*. NMC, London

CHAPTER I

The Mental Health Service User

James Dooher

Contemporary mental health nursing has its prime focus on the service user, their experience, their perceptions and their ability to meaningfully engage with the professional workforce in order to enhance their lives.

Service users are the fulcrum upon which the Multidisciplinary Team (MDT) and health providers operate, and all activity must be undertaken with the benefit of the service user in mind.

The terms 'service user', 'patient' and 'client' are interchangeably used within this book and within the broader literature base. Although the Department of Health (DH) and advocacy groups condone these terms, it is acknowledged that, these terms are not acceptable to all people: for example individuals who receive treatment against their will (Dooher and Byrt, 2003). However, it is difficult to find alternative terms which would be universally acceptable.

When considering the fundamental aspects of mental health nursing we must consider that, as nurses, everything we do and our whole reason for being, is for the patient. Without patients, mental health nurses do not exist, and it is this factor which must be held as a central tenet of the profession.

Historically this has not always been the case, but with rise of the service user movement, their voice is at last becoming increasingly louder, clearer and more articulate in the design, delivery and evaluation of mental health nursing. The prompt for change emanated from the government of the day, producing guidance in documents such as *Working for Patients* and *The Patient's Charter* (DH, 1989; DH, 1991). These aimed to improve the quality of health service delivery to patients, setting out patients' rights in the NHS and the standards of service they could expect to receive, including waiting times, information about services and treatment, and privacy and dignity. These documents established the *rights* (which all patients will receive all the time) and *expectations* (standards of service which the NHS is aiming to achieve), and set the agenda for the next two decades and hopefully beyond.

The Service User and Survivor Movement

In 2003, the Sainsbury Centre for Mental Health (SCMH) produced a policy paper (Wallcraft and Bryant, 2003) to identify and analyse organisations who represent adult users of mental health services across England. Their findings suggested that there were approximately 300 local service user groups who have common beliefs and understandings. This paper suggested that these binding factors constitute a movement rather than just a collection of separate organisations.

What constitutes the user/survivor movement is characteristically diverse and almost impossible to define (Mind, 2007). However the common beliefs understandings identified by SCMH, together with a desire to improve the experience for those who engage with mental health services, have drawn together individuals under a common purpose, and provided a universal platform on which to build articulate and informed alternative viewpoints. The spectrum of these views range from an abject anti-psychiatry lobby, for example those expressed by The Citizens Commission for Human Rights (CCHR), to those who work in partnership with, and for NHS Trusts such as the Patient Advocacy Liaison Groups (PALS).

Objections to the psychiatric system and treatment regimens have been noted throughout history and were not always welcome. These gathered momentum in the 1960s and began to become more coordinated in the 1970s with for example the Campaign Against Psychiatric Oppression and the development of diagnosis specific lobby groups such as the National Schizophrenia Fellowship (Now Rethink). In recent times this pluralistic diversity has been encouraged by successive Health Secretaries and has been underscored by key government documents. For example, the *National Service Framework for Mental Health* proposed that all mental health services must be planned and implemented in partnership with local communities and involve service users and carers (DH, 1999).

On the surface this appears to be a progressive and considered opportunity for individual service users and representative groups to influence both strategic policy and local implementation. However, we must be mindful that the political advantages to be gained from such involvement may lead to tokenism and the perfunctory inclusion of the users' view.

The degree of participation and its value to an organisational process or task can be considered in the light of Arnstein's Ladder, which identifies the levels of service user influence an organisation allows.

The factors which need to be considered in facilitating formal participation (and as a result service user empowerment), require a range of good practice and organisational maturity if true participation is to be achieved. Clear conceptualisation and ideas of what 'participation' means in relation to the service, and understanding of the desired degree and level of engagement are critical elements of a successful plan. Aims and goals should be specific and unambiguous, and supported by strategies, policies with target dates. These should be incorporated into an organisation's philosophy and mission statement. Clarity about whether empowerment/participation is an extrinsic goal, separate from other organisational goals; or intrinsic to some or all of these goals should form part of an organisation's self analysis. If empowerment/participation is extrinsic, clarity about its relative importance compared with other goals; and the extent that it complements or conflicts with them, will engender realism and indicate how achievable true participation will be.

The reciprocal need for participation was identified by Campbell (2005), who suggested that if independent action groups did not exist, there would be a need for the government to create something similar to replace them, and that the demand for involvement has a life of its own creating agendas over which service users may have limited control, and worryingly, that may not always serve their true interests.

There are a number of ways to help ensure the service user voice is heard, and clear communication from individual disciplines and managers will facilitate a more meaningful outcome. These may include: :

- Organisational self-awareness and reflection on previous practice and engagement
- Valuing service users/carers and their views and perspectives
- Positive, non – discriminatory attitudes and affirmation of identity, particularly of individuals stigmatised in wider society
- Active listening
- Facilitating appropriate platforms for the voice of service users and carers to be heard
- Taking individuals and their complaints and concerns seriously
- Providing opportunities for sharing information, engaging in consultation and collaborative projects

An organisation that listens to service users will facilitate the process at every level and be particularly mindful that at the epicentre of patient/professional communication is the therapeutic relationship. This may be seen as the primary agent of change in fulfilling the aims of personal growth. The Rogerian perspective (Rogers, 1951, 1959) suggests it is founded upon the therapist being genuine, congruent, empathetic, open, honest, non-judgmental and accepting of the client, and I propose that if an organisation can adopt the same stance, the likelihood of true participation will be greatly enhanced.

Changes to Thinking and Policy about Service Users

The Department of Health, relaunched the 10 High Impact Changes for Mental Health in 2006 (HICs) with the aim to improve quality of care and the efficiency of services, tailored to individual service user needs, and making the best use of resources to benefit service users (CSIP, NIMHE, 2006). The 10 High Impact Changes identify aspects of provision that could be improved and are suggested will improve the service users experience in the following ways:

- Less duplication
- Absence of 'ping-pong' effect
- Access to services closer to home
- Improved choice
- Better co-ordination of care
- Carer recognition
- Reduced delay in discharge
- Fewer delays shorter waiting times
- Less anxiety and greater satisfaction
- Clearer decision-making
- Greater control of self-care
- Information on where to get help
- Better quality of life.

The 10 High Impact Changes were developed by the Modernisation Agency based on their experience of implementing service improvement across the NHS. By implementing the 10 HICs systematically across the whole NHS, including primary, secondary and mental health settings, it is anticipated that patients will experience enhanced care delivery, which is more personalised, appropriate, timely and streamlined. That clinicians' hours, hospital bed days, and appointments in primary and secondary care will be saved, and clinical quality and clinical outcomes will be tangibly improved.

The very development of this document leads us to reflect that the aspirations of the Patient's Charter (DH, 1991) and succeeding efforts have not yet been realised, and that we should strive for a continual improvement. What can be said however, is that the HICs have an emphasis on efficiency and responsiveness to meet both local and national goals in addition to the change itself, and that as a direct outcome of implementing these measures, it will be easier to attract and retain staff, with a consequent increase in enjoyment and satisfaction at work. If the wellbeing of the workforce is assured then this should cascade into the wellbeing of the people who use services. The changes are:

1. Treat home-based care and support as the norm for the delivery of mental health services.

It is a long established fact that the 'home' is much preferred by service users and their carers as a place to receive their nursing care and treatment (Marks et al, 1994; Knapp et al, 1998; Fried et al, 1999, 2000; Leff et al, 2005). To underscore the research, the Department of Health suggests that:

> *'...wherever possible, patients must be able to make informed choices about treatment options, treatment providers, location for receiving care, and the type of ongoing care'.*

DH, 2005

Being nursed in ones' own home protects the individual from the debilitating effects of institutionalisation, and the inherent risks of being admitted into an environment that might further expose vulnerabilities. Although preferable, care based within the home is complex to organise, and influenced by many factors, needing careful planning, monitoring and evaluation if it is to be successful. This also means that inpatient services could well become providers for only a specialist or intensive type of service, making places hard to find for those who need one, and as an implicit consequence, people with more acute difficulties being treated for longer than acceptable periods in the community.

Explicit in the 10 High impact changes are the need for a greater provision for self help. This may take the shape of bibliotherapy (a book referral scheme) whereby by a list of self help books is made available across a county in public libraries and GP surgeries. This is seen as an effective empowering tool, which is difficult to overdose on and can be used whilst pregnant. It is also very cost-effective when compared to traditional consultation, referral and treatment pathways.

Hospital admission can be avoided when alternatives are in place such as day centres or other meaningful day time activity.

2. Improve flow of service users and carers across health and social care by improving access to screening and assessment.

Improving access to talking therapies for example counselling and psychology in primary care. Expert screening and assessment in primary care will enable service users to be either treated quickly whilst remaining in their own homes, signposted to the most appropriate facility or admitted into hospital.

However improved access to secondary care services may inhibited by the reduction of beds and resources that have been happening within primary care.

The complexity of introducing this type of service will necessitate improved referral guidelines and protocols, and better integrated health and mental health services.

3. Manage variation in service user discharge processes.

Timely and consistent discharge processes are needed to ensure service quality remains high no matter what day of the week a person leaves hospital. Critical to this outcome's success is the collaboration with service users and their carers in terms of being prepared for discharge, together with all the agencies that administer and facilitate the care programme approach.

4. Manage variation in access to all mental health services.

Developing responsive services that meet users' needs with a single point of access where appropriate, and consistent appointment booking processes which will improve the service users' experience. This will be achieved with better liaison and communication systems within primary care, accident and emergency departments, adult mental health, child and adolescent mental health, older peoples and criminal justice services.

Proactively managed systems will optimise clinician availability and improve the flow between health, mental health and other mainstream services.

5. Avoid unnecessary contact for service users and provide necessary contact in the right setting.

A commitment to delivering services with 'no needless delay' or 'no needless waste' has been echoed across the UK, and ensuring that appointments are effective is seen as one way of helping achieve that aspiration. The need for follow-up appointments should be a considered process and arise when there is either a clinical need, or at the request of the patient.

The efficiency savings afforded by this consideration will free up services for those who have a need. Where follow-up appointments are necessary, these should be provided in the right care setting and unnecessary follow-ups for patients will be avoided with a considered approach. Monitoring 'did not attend' (DNA) rates will be part of an organisation's evidence base. Effective caseload management, will reduce waste and facilitate a more efficient use of resources. This supports social inclusion of users in active rehabilitation and recovery.

6. Increase the reliability of interventions by designing care around what is known to work and that service users and carers inform and influence.

Increasing the reliability of therapeutic interventions through a care package approach where a number of scientifically proven measures or treatments are combined to improve recovery, and taking into consideration that the service user should be considered an expert in their own symptoms, relapse signatures and care will enable a greater influence in the treatment regimes. Service users and carers should be at the centre of decision-making and establish systems that support meaningful service user and carer involvement and participation (Dooher and Byrt, 2003).

7. Apply a systematic approach to enable the recovery of people with long term conditions.

The notion of recovery is a possibility for those with enduring and severe mental health problems was emphasised in the 2001 document *The Journey to Recovery,* the government's vision for mental health care (DH, 2001), in that there is a recognition for the whole mental health system to support people in settings of their own choosing, enabling access to community resources including housing, education, work, friendships — or whatever *they* think is critical to their own recovery. The High Impact Changes promote an approach that supports and empowers people with long term conditions to better manage their mental health.

Copeland (1997, 2004) considered a number of essential elements for effective recovery work:

- Instilling hope and the notion that people who experience mental health difficulties do get well, stay well and go on to meet their life dreams and goals, thus achieving their personal optimum potential
- Promoting personal responsibility for the patient to acknowledge that their own efforts are a key part of becoming well and with the assistance of others, taking action and do what needs to be done to keep well.
- Empowerment through education where learning about the illness or symptoms can better promote informed decision making
- Self Advocacy and effectively reaching out to others to secure what is wanted, needed, and deserved to support wellbeing and recovery.
- Recognition that to enhance ones quality of life interdependence with those around us and their support will be needed.

8. Improve service user flow by removing queues.

Waiting for treatment for any health condition can promote anxiety and impact on the eventual prognosis of the issue. Waiting for treatment in mental health is particularly distressing for both the patient and their families. The aim of this target is to reduce the time service users wait at any point in the health and social care process, for example between referral and the first appointment and any referrals to internal services.

The *Depression Report* (Layard, 2006) advocates increasing access to psychological therapies, especially Cognitive Behaviour Therapy (CBT) in order to help alleviate the suffering of people with mental health problems. It suggests that psychological therapies, particularly CBT, should be made available to people suffering from depression, chronic anxiety and schizophrenia. It estimates that 10,000 new therapists will be needed by 2013 to treat an estimated 800,000 to one million at-risk individuals every year through the creation of 250 treatment centres, each comprising between 20 and 40 therapists. The report puts forward the idea that depression and chronic anxiety are the biggest causes of misery in Britain today, and laments this 'waste of people's lives'.

The reality for patients seeking therapy is that they often have little choice, because there are too few appropriately trained therapists and it could be said that the recommendation of CBT will further limit their choice as it is not a panacea for all problems. There is however a strong evidence base for CBT but as a single recommended approach it limits the opportunity to access a range of alternatives, such as person-centred approaches, and other forms of psychotherapy. Where CBT comes into its own is that it is time based and reasonably cheap to deliver .

Lack of access, issues of stigma, and poor recognition of psychological disorders in primary care mean that the prevalence of untreated mental health problems in the community is high.

The major barrier to this development is a shortage of therapists and a requirement for major organisational change if the programme is to be delivered. Teams will usually lead by a clinical psychologist, and be comprised of individuals from a range of professional backgrounds, nurses, OTs, social workers for example, all trained in CBT.

9. Optimise service user and carer flow through the service using an integrated care pathway approach.

Integrated Care Pathways (ICPs) outline the optiimal course of care for all patients with a specific disorder, and are founded upon a contemporary evidence base. It is suggested that they increase efficiency and outcomes through a whole service systematic approach to delivering a care package and relies on input from multidisciplinary teams. The multidisciplinary team considers the optimal sequence and timing of interventions, and because pathways traverse different disciplines/health districts, they help ensure that coordinated quality services are provided over the full continuum of care. ICPs can minimise delays and make best use of resources and have the potential to assist in completion of a single assessment and care plan. Cross disciplinary working with communal notes improves communication which is particularly useful for discharge planning and the Care Programme Approach (CPA), help information flow between care settings, professionals and districts, and must be informative to service users.

ICPs optimise patient flow through service bottlenecks using process templates and as health and social care organisations respond to the health modernisation agenda, the use of integrated care pathways in mental health is becoming a universally accepted process. Hall and Howard's (2006) *Care Pathways* detail expected multidisciplinary interventions within a care experience and use variances to monitor care and facilitate quality improvement have been emerging throughout UK mental health services over the last few years.

10. Redesign and extend roles in line with efficient service user and carer pathways to attract and retain an effective workforce (CSIP, 2006).
There is now a clear body of evidence-based best practice, which improve the patient experience, and the efficiency of health services but to enable that evidence to be translated into an improved experience for the patient, then consideration needs to be given to the skills expertise and professional disposition of the staff. This change aims to ensure that the services provided meet the needs of service users and carers and that skilled and motivated staff are recruited and retained.

The demands placed upon the mental health nursing workforce and the multidisciplinary team develop in both evolutionary and revolutionary ways and ensuring that the skills of the workforce are consistent with service need and the delivery of a patient-focused service is the key feature of workforce planning and development.

The redesign of roles enables the workforce to be responsive to new demands and improves the likelihood that workers are fit for purpose. This should reduce fragmentation and role demarcation and at the same time

---

Learning Points

1. As nurses, everything we do, and our whole reason for being, is for the patient. Without patients, mental health nurses do not exist, and it is this factor which must be held as a central tenet of the profession.
2. If organisations are genuine, congruent, empathetic, open, honest, non-judgmental and accepting of the client, the likelihood of true participation will be greatly enhanced.
3. The 10 High Impact Changes aim to improve quality of care and the efficiency of services, tailored to individual service user needs, and making the best use of resources to benefit service users.

shape previously Inflexible career structures. Role redesign identifies levels of skill and how these might fit into a broader service redesign. This may improve career paths, and through training, education and professional regulation ensure that workers are fit for practice and purpose.

The Department of Health suggest that nursing is changing almost as rapidly as the context in which it is practised and that role redesign will enable improved efficiencies, faster response times, more effective use of time, better continuity of care and removal of barriers. They suggest nursing is adapting to meet the needs of patients and the public, and nurses have taken on new roles, work across boundaries, and are setting up new services to meet patients' needs (DH, 2006).

References

Arnstein S (1969) *A Ladder of Citizen Participation*. American Institute of Planners, Washington DC: No 3 (Part 4) 216.

Campbell P (2005) *Beyond the Water Towers The unfinished revolution in mental health services 1985-2005*. The Sainsbury Centre for Mental Health, London

Copeland ME (1997) *Wellness Recovery Action Plan*. Peach Press, Dummerston, VT

Copeland ME (2004) Self-determination in mental health recovery: Taking back our lives. In: Jonikas J, Cook J, eds. *UIC NRTC's National Self-Determination and Psychiatric Disability Invitational Conference: Conference Papers*. UIC National Research and Training Centre on Psychiatric Disability, Chicago, IL

CSIP, NIMHE (2006) *10 High Impact Changes for Mental Health Services*. Department of Health, London

Dooher J, Byrt R (2002) *Empowerment and Participation: Power influence and control in contemporary healthcare*. volume 1. Quay Books, London

Dooher J, Byrt R (2003) *Empowerment and the Health Service User*. Quay Books, London

DH (1989) *Working for Patients*. HMSO, London

DH (1991) *The Patient's Charter*. Department of Health, London

DH (1999) *National Service Framework for Mental Health Modern Standards and Service Models*. Department of Health, London

DH (2005) *Creating a patient-led NHS: Delivering the NHS Improvement Plan*. Department of Health, London

DH (2006) *Modernising Nursing Careers – Setting the Direction*. Department of Health, London

Fried TR, Doorn C, O'Leary JR, Tinetti ME, Drickamer MA (1999) Older persons' perceptions of home and hospital as sites of treatment for acute illness. *Am J Med* **107**:

317-23

Fried TR, van Doorn C, O'Leary JR, Tinetti ME, Drickamer MA (2000) Older persons' preferences for home vs hospital care in the treatment of acute illness. *Arch Intern Med* **160**: 1501-6

Knapp M, Marks I, Woolstenholme J, Beecham J,Astin J, Audini B, Connolly J, Watts V (1998) Home-based versus hospital-based care for serious mental illness. Controlled cost-effectiveness study over four years. *British Journal of Psychiatry* **172**: 506-12

Hall J, Howard D, (2006) *Integrated Care Pathways in Mental Health* Churchill Livingstone, London

Layard R (2006) *The Depression Report.* London School of Economics' Centre for Economic Performance Mental Health Policy Group, London

Leff B, Burton L, Mader SL,Naughton B, Burl J, Inouye SK, Greenough III SB, Guido S,Langston C, Frick KD, Steinwachs D, and Burton JR (2005) Hospital at Home: Feasibility and Outcomes of a Program To Provide Hospital-Level Care at Home for Acutely Ill Older Patients. *Annals of Internal Medicine* **143**: 798-808

Marks IM, Connolly J, Muijen M, Audini B, McNamee G and Lawrence RE (1994) Home-based versus hospital-based care for people with serious mental illness. *British Journal of Psychiatry* **165**: 179-194

Mind (2007) LOCN *Mind Information Volunteer Training Course; Module 2 Private Study Materials.* Mind, London

Rogers CR (1959) A theory of therapy, personality and interpersonal relationships as developed in the client-centered framework. In: Koch, S, ed. *Psychology: A study of a science. Vol. III. Formulations of the person and the social context.* McGraw Hill, New York

Rogers CR (1951) *Client-centered Therapy: Its Current Practice, Implications and Theory.* Houghton Mifflin, Boston

Wallcraft J, Bryant M (2003) *Policy Paper 2, The Mental Health Service User Movement In England.* The Sainsbury Centre for Mental Health, London

CHAPTER 2

Quality and Mental Health Nursing

Kelvin Ford

This chapter provides an overview of the concept of quality, including its inception in the manufacturing industry, and includes an overview of the concept of quality within the health service. Quality protocols arising from the manufacturing industry have been adopted by the health service, particularly since the 1980s, and an historical overview describes the different policy changes which has influenced its application. Several quality methods are currently used in mental health services, including standard setting, direct action, creating a quality system, professional/clinical audit, total quality management, consumer feedback and quality monitoring tools.

This overview is not exhaustive and attempts to summarise some of the most salient elements of developing and maintaining quality in mental health care.

Developing, Maintaining and Reviewing Quality in Mental Health

The Concept of Quality

There are many definitions of quality. At its most basic, quality may be defined as a degree or the level of excellence. However, within the health service it would be a mistake to assume that it is underpinned by common understandings of quality, for definitions of quality vary between different groups.

The concept of quality originated initially from the manufacturing industry. The 1920s saw the introduction of formal quality control systems, which introduced control charts and statistical processes. This development was an attempt to move from inspection processes specifically designed to identify and remove faulty products during production, to controls aimed at increasing the number of good products being manufactured. The so-called 'Plan-Do-Check-Act' forms the foundation of most quality systems today (Joss and Kogan, 1995). Indeed, manufacturers who could not compete in terms of quality and value for money soon collapsed as a business. It was in the best interests for all concerned to invest, develop and maintain quality control.

During the late 1940s the philosophy changed from quality control to quality assurance. This resulted in more emphasis on pre-production planning, where attempts were made to systematically design out errors during production. Indeed, it became apparent that most errors could be attributed to process design. This development was termed the 'quality revolution' and is believed to have been introduced initially in the Japanese manufacturing industry during the 1950s. However, the concept of quality assurance requires its workers to adopt a 'quality culture' and therefore to take ownership of quality (Joss and Kogan, 1995).

Over the past 80 years the concept of quality has been developed by several organisations, using a number of approaches, some of which are theoretically underpinned, whilst others are not.

Quality in Health Care

Quality in health care can be defined in different ways. Clinicians, for example, may focus on 'doing the right thing for the right people at the right time' (Donaldson and Gray, 1998). Patients, on the other hand, 'do not feel qualified to judge technical quality — they assess their health care by other dimensions which reflect what they personally value' (Kenagy et al, 1999).

According to Ovretveit (1992), the aim of quality assurance has been to provide the highest standards of care within available resources, whilst ensuring good value for the taxpayer. Continual improvement in health care comes from giving people new methods and skills to analyse the quality problems, issues and processes, and by empowering them to make any necessary changes and improvements. It does not come from relying solely on inspections and standard-setting and exhaustive customer relations training. This is very significant, for, in many cases, staff providing the care are often in the best position to identify quality problems and to suggest ways of solving and improving these and to build on existing strengths and good practice.

However, although demand for mental health care appears to be increasing, funding does not necessarily keep in step. Indeed, some mental health units are currently facing closure due to overspending or under-funding problems. Clearly, the availability of financial and human resources is an important issue effecting the quality of mental health care (Shepard et al, 2002).

Inevitably, developing and maintaining quality assurance in mental health care puts extra pressures of work on staff. Therefore, what is the incentive for staff? Improving and maintaining a quality health service can increase job satisfaction, may result in less complaints, improve recruitment and retention and reduce negligence and compensation claims.

Ovretveit (1992) suggests that a quality health service is one which recognises three dimensions:

- **Client quality** (what clients and carers want from the service)
- **Professional quality** (whether the service meets the needs as defined by professional providers, and whether it carries out techniques and procedures which are necessary to meet client needs)
- **Management quality** (the most efficient and productive use of resources, within the limits and directives set by higher authorities or commissioners).

The Development of Quality Assurance Within the Health Service

When the NHS was introduced in 1948 there was no particular agenda for quality. Indeed, it was taken for granted that appropriate quality would arise from the provision of an infrastructure and would result in training and education of appropriate staff (Nicholls et al, 2000). Although efforts were made over the next two decades to develop quality improvements, this tended to focus on rearranging tangible components of the health service such as developing more and better equipment, updating buildings and facilities, plus training and education of staff. However, because these developments were separately apportioned, it was inevitable that a lack of 'connectedness' became apparent, resulting in inefficiency, duplication and the generation of complicated processes.

During the 1970s, both analysts and thinkers attempted to define and explain the meaning and relevance of components of quality, including standards, criteria and norm, for example. This in turn gave rise to the importance of understanding the relationship between structures, processes and outcomes (Nichols et al, 2000).

In the UK, further impetus to measure quality in the health service came from Conservative governments during the 1980s, with the Griffiths Report (1993) recommending that quality assurance should be an integral part of the evaluation and provision of services, with particular attention given to the views and expressed needs of patients (DHSS, 1983). Five years later, a survey by the National Association of Health Authorities revealed at least eighty schemes for improving the responsiveness of the NHS to the needs of its consumers (TRHA, 1988). Guidelines on quality assurance and the monitoring of services were initially addressed in the Community Care Act (1990). In addition, in 1990 the Department of Health and the former UKCC (now the NMC) have both stated that nurses must become more accountable for their practice (DH, 1990; UKCC, 1989). This increased accountability and involves, in part, the development of standards of nursing care based on careful assessment and evaluations by both clients and staff.

During the 1990s managers became accountable for output measures and targets were created in '*Health of the Nation*' (DH, 1992) and '*Our Healthier Nation*' (DH, 1998). However, according to Nichols et al (2000), these targets related to financial and workload concerns, and thus 'cost containment' became an increasing problem in a service which was demand-led. During this decade too there was increasing consensus that improved use of evidence-based research would result in improved outcomes and consistency of approach. '*A Modern and Dependable NHS*' (DH, 1997) focused on the issue of health care quality. Quality in the health service, therefore, became a 'prevailing purpose rather than a desirable accessory'. The government had introduced for the first time a statutory duty regarding quality and introduced the concept of corporate governance, which previously had only been relevant to financial and workload issues.

In 1998, clinical governance policy was introduced. The term 'clinical governance' is used to describe the framework through which health organisations are accountable for continuously improving the quality of their services and safeguarding high standards of care. It has become the main vehicle for continuously improving the quality of client care (Arya and Callaly, 2005). According to Nicholls et al (2000), clinical governance can be viewed as a whole system cultural change which facilitates the process of developing the organisational capability to deliver sustainable, accountable, patient-focused quality assured health care. Implementing a clinical governance framework successfully also requires clear clinical leadership, the development of structures and processes to facilitate communication, and the development of systems for monitoring and evaluating mental health services (Arya and Callaly, 2005).

The National Institute for Clinical Excellence (NICE) was introduced in 1999 to provide national guidance on the promotion of good health and the prevention and treatment of ill health. NICE has since joined with the Health Development Agency to become the New National Institute for Clinical Excellence (NICE, 2006).

The Commission for Health Improvement (CHI) formed in 2000 also formed part of a structured response at a national level in order to ensure quality improvement in health care (Nicholls et al, 2000).

In 2005, the Department of Health commissioned a team specifically to focus on quality outcome measures in mental health care. The resulting outcome measures are broad and include: measurement, monitoring of data, treatment management, and benchmarking (Fonagy et al, 2005). It is expected that the document will help Trusts in developing an approach to outcome measures that will facilitate the healthcare commission along with the implementation of their own benchmarking initiatives. Highlighted in the report is the vital role of 'front line staff' in the use and development of these outcome measures

Clearly, the concept of quality in health care has gradually developed over the last few decades and now features high on the health service agenda. However, in order to introduce and maintain a quality programme in mental health and social care, organisations need to plan and develop a quality framework. This involves a combination of quality methods and controls. Relying on just one method for maintaining a quality service will not suffice. Using several quality methods, therefore, provides a much wider and accurate picture of the overall quality.

Setting Standards

The first place to begin is to formulate a set of quality standards. A standard relates to a specific expectation by staff. This may include a particular activity or outcome which can be measured and is specified in relation to a level of performance to be achieved within a defined measure or indicator (Ovretveit, 1992).

Standards should be achievable, measurable and clear. Where possible staff involved in achieving a particular standard should be involved in setting the standard as opposed to a 'top down' management approach, thus creating a sense of ownership. Service users can also be involved in setting standards, thereby providing a different perspective. The effectiveness of standard setting can be improved through training and by providing information and literature for staff.

Once the quality of care is defined as a set of standards, the mental health service can be measured. A comparison can be made against what is currently happening to that which is intended. It is common practice to select several standards to measure on a regular routine basis, and to select other standards which are more broader which can usually be measured annually.

In the current climate, staff need to provide evidence of what they do. Indeed, if, for example, a standard states that each client will have an individual care plan which is evaluated at least on a weekly basis, then relevant staff need to provide evidence for this.

Taking Direct Action

The health service is a largely a labour-intensive service and thus depends on people to provide a care service, as opposed to relying on machines, robots or computers. Every person working in an organisation has responsibility for quality — from the chief executive to the cleaners; it is a collective responsibility. Even a small item such as answering the telephone can create a good or bad impression.

Quality problems and potential problems can occur on a daily basis and it is up to staff to address these problems, as soon as practicable, in order to prevent an escalation. In many cases, this requires common sense and can usually be addressed within a short period during the course of work. Quality problems and issues can also be raised as a result of complaints or highlighted by staff, clients or stakeholders. In many cases, staff, are in the best position to find solutions to the problem.

According to Ovretveit (1992), where quality performance is perceived as poor, a subject is picked for corrective action. Quality methods can be used to select which subject to focus on. Focus or quality group meetings can be organised to discuss possible causes and to decide what changes to make. Action plans can then be created in order to address the problem, which in turn would need an evaluation of the results to prevent a re-occurrence.

Creating a Quality System

A quality system involves the roles and responsibilities, procedures and processes which an organisation needs to ensure that staff are able to provide the care required. One of the key aims of a quality system is to enhance the way quality is improved and to make changes, as necessary, in order to allow the service to function better. There is an assumption that the cost of a quality system is offset by the savings. Indeed, some purchasers will only provide contracts with provider units when a sound quality system is in place (Ovretveit, 1992).

Professional and Clinical Audit

One method of improving quality in mental health care is by each professional group conducting an audit. Although most experience with the audit process is contained within a particular profession, in many mental health care settings health and social care professionals work within a multidisciplinary team and therefore require multidisciplinary solutions to problems. Each professional group should include methods of noting and addressing quality issues which involves other professions, and inter-professional quality problems can be addressed by liaison members within audit groups. In many cases nursing and medical staff review their practice in postgraduate training, case presentation and ward rounds, for example. Both these formal and informal encounters primarily focus on individual cases as opposed to utilising systematic techniques to facilitate mental health service improvements, which are designed and evaluated accordingly.

In contrast, an audit uses scientific or systematic methods to create specific criteria for good practice, measure performance, compare results with peers, select cases, and to decide and introduce improvements. The process also involves the recording of the audit process and to quantify and present the results (Ovretveit, 1992).

Audit requires that professionals must decide what constitutes best practice, outcome criteria, indicators and how to conduct assessments and treatments. The process ultimately involves why there are variations from best practice and to identify what improvements can be made. The process then involves follow-up and evaluation to identify whether improvements have been made and whether they were effective. The main aim of the audit process, therefore, is to increase professionals understanding of the health care delivery, where quality problems occur, and the areas in which they need to make efforts to avoid problems (Ovretveit, 1992).

Melvin et al (2005), for example, conducted an audit focusing on the quality of inpatient care before and after service redesign. This audit examined the number of incidents, the number of days the wards were locked, observation levels, sickness and the number of bank hours used. The results showed that the rates of these factors did not increase following redesign.

Total Quality Management

When healthcare staff have received appropriate training and experience in quality methods and procedures, it is appropriate to consider Total Quality Management (TQM). Joss and Kogan (1995) define TQM as 'an integrated, corporately led programme of organisational change designed to engender and sustain a culture of continuous improvement based on customer-orientated definitions of quality'.

One of the problems with quality assurance is that it has limitations regarding the extent to which a group of workers can influence change. Indeed, one limitation within industry was that early problem-solving teams consisted of mainly intra-departmental and uni-disciplinary workers. Since many services span inter-departmental boundaries, workers found that they had little influence on materials and personnel. Moreover, it was found that the overwhelming majority of actual improvements required changes in policy or cross-functional practice that were traditionally the responsibility of managers. The result was a widening of quality assurance in order to take into account all those activities within the organisation and to extend the process of quality assurance to the organisation's external stakeholders. Programmes thus became increasingly corporate and top-down in perspective. In turn, statements began to appear in the organisation's mission statements and quality protocols featured as part of the normal business planning process (Joss and Kogan, 1995).

TQM takes the quality approach a step further and attempts to ensure that all health workers practise the methods and philosophy of quality assurance. It is essential, however, that a quality system is in place before TQM is introduced (Ovretveit, 1992).

Consumer Satisfaction Studies and Consumer Feedback

The notion of involving clients and the public in health care planning and delivery has been on the agenda for several years. In practice, most health organisations could offer evidence that they have consulted the public on the latest plans for service development, and most clinicians would believe that client involvement occurs on every occasion in the interview room. However, for many healthcare workers, the leap may not necessary be made to the underlying rationale for involvement, which is to develop a partnership that enables dialogue regarding choices, which in turn, leads to the best possible experience of health care (Squire et al, 2006; DH, 2004)

According to Squire et al (2006), organisational and professional structures often militate against the development of this consumer involvement in health care. One of the biggest challenges, therefore, is to ensure that the organisational and team cultures that surround the relationship between client and health professional actively support the principles of partnership. Indeed, in our research study, several general practitioners, in particular, felt that patient involvement in health care was 'dangerous' and 'inappropriate' (Ford et al, 1997).

Health cultures, therefore, need to continue to nurture the practice of engagement with clients and carers for all health professionals in their training and continuing professional education and practice.

Research studies highlight that consumers of health care can provide a useful source of information which can highlight both the positive and negative aspects of mental health care and may add a perspective that health professionals may not appreciate. These studies have used a variety of research methods, particularly questionnaires and semi-structured interviewing and focus groups (e.g. Lammers and Happell, 2004; Ford et al, 1999; Farrell, 2004; Scheyett et al, 2006). It must also be noted, however, that clients' may not necessarily be aware of their needs or quality problems that effect them. Furthermore, they may not necessarily be able to articulate their true opinions due to their mental health problem or for fear that criticism may be held against them (despite assurances to the contrary).

A number of people have written about their experiences as users of mental health services (Robins et al, 2005), whilst others have started or joined voluntary organisations to provide mutual support and in some cases, to protest at the way they have been devalued or badly treated. Partly, in response to this movement, some professionals have attempted to empower clients and enable their participation in their care and treatment. In addition several bodies have been concerned with the monitoring of quality in mental health services, including the Mental Health Act Commission, Health Advisory Service, MIND and other voluntary organisations.

Over the past two decades there has been increased interest in clients' perceptions of care, their rights and the role of nurses as both advocate and facilitators of client empowerment and participation in their care. One way to facilitate the process of participation is the systematic collection of clients' views about their care and the use of these views to effect improvements.

Quality Monitoring Tools

Aspects of quality assurance includes an evaluation of existing care and regular monitoring to ensure that high standards are achieved and maintained. Quality assurance is also concerned with highlighting examples of good practice and the sharing of these practices. A quality tool can provide an aid to systematically identifying, analysing and resolving quality problems.

Many quality monitoring tools have largely proved their worth in a variety of organisations and have since been adapted and applied within the health service. Although a certain amount of training is often advised before use, a high degree of skill is usually not necessary (Ovretveit, 1992).

A study conducted by Valenstein et al (2004) examined mental health provider's perceptions of monitoring mental health services. Most mental health care providers (65%) felt that quality-monitoring tools could be valuable in efforts to improve care. However, only 38% felt able to influence performance related to these monitors. Providers were most positive about satisfaction monitors. Despite providers' relatively positive views of monitors, 41% felt that monitoring programmes did not assist them in improving care.

A variety of tools to monitor and measure the quality of mental health care are currently on the market. However, it is important not to rush out and apply just any monitoring tool, as each one focuses on different aspects of mental health care and time is needed to decide what precisely is required to be measured.

Although produced several years ago, both *Quartz* (Clifford et al, 1989) and *Psychiatric Monitor* (Goldstone and Hunter, 1985) are currently used to monitor general aspects of mental health care. Others have been designed for particular aspects of mental health care.

Durbin et al (2003), for example, produced a monitoring tool to measure status and outcome of clients' using mental health outpatient and community programmes, the results of which provided a core of information to which measurement of more in-depth issues could be addressed.

Hodges and Wotring (2004) produced a monitoring tool to monitor the outcomes of youths with serious emotional disturbances who are treated in the public sector. Additional reports were used to ensure record compliance, monitor at-risk youths and assist in reviewing the adequacy of treatment plans. The consistently poor outcomes for some types of clients' generated an interest among clinical staff in learning and implementing evidence-based treatments.

Learning Points

1. Quality control, and later quality assurance, originated initially within the manufacturing industry
2. Quality assurance was subsequently adopted by the NHS mainly in the 1980s in response to policy changes
4. Mental health services should design and invest in a quality framework, which meets the needs of its consumers and stakeholders, within resource limitations
5. A quality framework would usually include the following methods: standard setting; taking direct action; quality control system; professional audit; total quality management; and consumer feedback quality monitoring tools.

References

Arya D, Callaby T (2005) Using Continuous Quality Improvement to Implement a Clinical Governance Framework in a Mental Health Service. *Health Service Journal* **13**(3): 241-6

Clifford P, Leiper R, Lavender A, Pillings S (1989) *Assuring Quality in Mental Health Services. The Quartz System.* Free Association Books, London.

DH (1990) *Caring for Patients.* DH, London

DH (1992) *The Health of the Nation.* HMSO, London

DH (1998) *Our Healthier Nation.* DoH, London

DH and Social Security (1983) *NHS Management Enquiry Report (the Griffiths Report).* HMSO; London

DH (2004) *The NHS Improvement Plan: Putting People at the Heart of Public Services, Cm 6268.* HMSO, London

Donaldson L, Gray J (1998) Clinical Governance: A Quality Duty for Health Organisations. *Quality in Health Care* **7**: 537–44

Durbin J, Prendergast P, Dewa CS, Rush B, Cooke RG (2003) Mental Health Programme Monitoring: Towards simplifying a complex task. *Psychiatric Rehabilitation* **26**(3): 249-61

Farrell C (2004) *Patient and Public Involvement in Health: The evidence for policy implementation*. DH, London

Fonagy P, Mathews R, Pilling S (2005) *Outcome Measures Implementation Best Practice Guidance*. DH, Leeds

Ford K, Middleton J, Palmer R, Farrington A (1997) Primary Health Care workers Training Needs in Mental Health. *British Journal of Nursing* **6**(21): 1244-1250

Ford KG, Sweeney J, Farrington A (1999) User Views of a Regional Secure Unit – Findings From A Patient Satisfaction Study. *International Journal of Psychiatric Nursing Research* 5,(1): 526–541

Goldstone C, Hunter D (1985) *Psychiatric Monitor*. Scutari

Hodges K, Wotring J (2004) The Role of Monitoring Outcomes in Initiating Implementation of Evidence-based Treatments at the State Level. *Psychiatric Service* 55(4): 396-400

Joss R, Kogan M (1995) *Advancing Quality: Total Quality Management in the National Health Service. Chapter one*. Open University Press, Buckingham

Kenagy JW, Berwick DM, Shore MF (1999) Service Quality in Health Care. *JAMA* **281**(7): 661-5

Lammers J, Happell B (2004) Research Involving Mental Health Consumers and Carers: a reference group approach. *International Journal of Mental Health Nursing* **13**(4): 262-6

Melvin M, Hall P, Bienck E (2005) Redesigning Acute Mental Health Services: An audit into the quality of inpatient care before and after service redesign in Grampian. *Psychiatric Mental Health Nursing* **12**(6): 733-8

Nichols S, Cullen R, O'Neill S, Halligan A (2000) Clinical Governance its Origins and its Foundations. *Clinical Performance and Quality Health Care* **8**(3): 172-178

Ovretveit J (1992) *Health Service Quality: An introduction to Quality Methods for Health Services. Chapter one*. Blackwell, London

Robins CS, Sauvageot JA, Cusack KJ, Suffoletta-Maierle and Fruch BC (2005) Consumers Perceptions of Negative Experiences and 'Sanctuary Harm' in Psychiatric Settings. *Psychiatric Service* **56**(12): 1622-25

Scally G, Donaldson LJ (1998) Looking Forward: Clinical Governance and the Drive for Quality Improvement in the New NHS in England. *British Medical Journal* **317**(7150): 61-5

Scheyett A, McCarthy E, Rausch C (2006) Consumer and Family Views on Evidence-Based Practices and Adult Mental Health Services. *Community Mental Health Journal* 13th March

Secretary of State for Health (1997) *The New NHS: Modern and Dependable*. HMSO, London

Shepard DS, Daley M, Ritter GA, Hodgkin D, Beinecke RH (2002) Managed Care and the Quality of Substance Abuse Treatment. *Mental Health Policy Economics* **5**(4): 163-74

Squire S, Greco M, O'Hagan B, Dickinson K, Wall D (2006) Being Patient-Centred: Creating health care for our grandchildren. *Clinical Governance International Journal* **11**(1): 8-16

Trent Regional Health Authority (1998) *From Me to You. A Management Process to Achieve a Personalised Service.* TRHA, Sheffield

UKCC (1989) *Exercising Accountability.* UKCC, London

Valenstein M, Mitchinson A, Ronis DL, Alexander JA, Duffy SA, Craig TJ, Barry KL (2004) Quality Indicators and Monitoring of Mental Health Services: What do frontline providers think? *American Journal of Psychiatry* **161**(1): 146-53

CHAPTER 3

The Multidisciplinary Team

James Dooher

There are many different professional groups involved in the assessment, planning, implementation and evaluation of mental health care. Collectively they are described as the Multidisciplinary Team (MDT). This chapter will describe some of the roles and responsibilities of the individual professions involved in the delivery of mental health care.

There are many definitions of what a team is and does, but Mohrman et al (1995) capture the essence of a team in their description of a group of individuals who work together to produce products or deliver services for which they take collective responsibility. They suggest that team members share goals, and are mutually held accountable for meeting them, and that results are shaped by their interactions with one another. As the team is held collectively accountable, the work of integrating with one another is included among the responsibilities of each individual member and this encourages individual effort from each member, hopefully producing a better outcome than if the individuals were to work independently.

The terms 'multidisciplinary', 'interdisciplinary' and 'interprofessional' are often used interchangeably, and although there is some debate about the differences between these groupings, for the purposes of this chapter and ease of understanding we will assume that they are all the same. This said, there have been a number of Government policies (DH, 1997, 1998; NHSE, 1999; CHI, 2004) that advocate multidisciplinary, interprofessional and interdisciplinary working as a means of achieving the new agenda in the NHS. These policies share the vocabulary of collaboration, and highlight a shift from what has been described as 'uniprofessional' working, where activities of professions are confined within their own discipline, and 'multiprofessionalism', where professions recognise that other disciplines have an important contribution to make. However they promote the notion of interprofessional working, which is where practitioners are said to make a commitment to work with each other across boundaries for the benefit of the patient or client (Freeman et al, 2000).

One of the key aspects of professional development is achieved through and by reflecting on their practice (Schon, 1983), a process which is covered elsewhere in this book, but it is the notion of interdependence and shared purpose which binds and protects individual members of an MDT.

It has been suggested that there are significant advantages of team working for team members. Borrill et al (2000) suggest that people who work in teams are much clearer about what their jobs entail because team working enables good communication and detailed negotiation of effective work roles. Those working in teams also report a high level of social support, both practically and emotionally, during times of difficulty or stress. As a consequence, working in a team enables employees to be protected from the stress that many feel within the NHS. Borrill et al (2000) go on to promote the idea that NHS employees working in a team perceive that there is generally more co-operation in the organisation than others who do not work in a team, leading to more positive work attitudes, and are more likely co-operate with others within the organisation. They also suggest that team membership buffers individuals from the effects of negative organisational climate and conflict.

Teamwork and effective communication are essential to the success of most businesses and organizations, and it is important for the mental health nurse to recognise the significance of team working in the delivery of high quality care. The promotion, maintenance and restoration of health care requires a diverse range of people, each with their individual ideas,

Characteristics of High Performing Teams

1. Share a common purpose or set of goals
2. Communicate effectively
3. Practice effective dialogue instead of debate, and identify and resolve group conflicts
4. Encourage transparency in how problems are solved and decisions are made, build relationships that promote trust, respect and empathy
5. Plan thoroughly before acting, but review the plan regularly and consistently
6. Balance the task that needs to be achieved and the process or means by which it is achieved
7. Respect and value each others' 'diversity' and vary levels and intensity of work, providing a balance between work and home
8. Reward and value individual performance that supports the team
9. Promote and support team goals, acknowledging the interdependence required to meet them
10. Critically evaluate working practice and methods to improve quality.

philosophies, history and methods of care. They are required to work closely together, and this closeness can sometimes lead to tension and conflict, which may impact team performances (West et al, 2003). Many nurses might say that they work in teams, but surveys have found that many of these 'teams' lack structure and, therefore, leadership (CHI, 2004), which is a critical factor for teams to be effective (Zaccaro et al, 2000). Mental health nurses can provide strong leadership through the development of their knowledge and skills, which in turn improves patient confidence and relationships.

Carter et al (2003) suggest that when patients know that they are being looked after by a team they get a sense of assurance similar to that of having a second opinion, reducing the fear that their treatment is based on the knowledge of just one clinician. They propose that it is easier to provide continuity of good quality care with multidisciplinary team working, and that shared clinical responsibility for patients shares the stress of those who provide it.

Team working provides an opportunity for more effective communication and enhances opportunities to speak directly to each other about clinical matters. Discussing the care of individual patients allows the sharing of ideas which would not be apparent in one-on-one clinical encounters. Team working increases the sense of partnership and provides friendship and support, particularly in difficult clinical situations such as the management of clinical errors and complaints. Sharing of knowledge becomes easier, and the collective power of the MDT may improve chances of arguing effectively for more resources.

Team Roles

The Role of the Social Worker

Traditionally, there are two main types of social worker in mental health work: the social worker (SW) and the approved social worker (ASW). They are both members of the multidisciplinary team and in the main employed by a local authority. They may be involved in a number of ways and work in a variety of settings.

Social workers offer advice on practical matters, financial support such as welfare benefits, day care and accommodation, or provide a link between different services. Some social workers are trained in mental health and can offer counselling. Hospital social workers are attached to both general and psychiatric hospitals. A 'psychiatric social worker' is a specialist who works closely with individuals and families to support them either through crises or in the longer term.

An ASW is a qualified social worker who has undergone additional training and has been approved by the local authority to carry out designated functions under the Mental Health Act 1983. An ASW has a role in mental health assessment under the Act, undertaken jointly with other medical professionals, and provides a perspective on compulsory admission to hospital. ASWs have a particular responsibility to examine alternatives to hospitalisation and enable the patient to remain in their community (in conjunction with mental health nurses).

Social workers and ASWs are facing fundamental changes to their role, with staff being seconded to, or employed directly by NHS Trusts, and a pressure to move away from generalist or generic social workers to specialist teams, including a specific mental health service.

The proposed changes in the Mental Health Bill (to be implemented in October 2008) provide an additional catalyst for change, where the role of the ASW will be undertaken by an approved mental health practitioner (AMHP), who may, or may not, have a social work background.

When it becomes law, the new Mental Health Act will allow for a broadening of the groups of practitioners that are able to fulfil functions currently undertaken by Approved Social Workers (ASWs) and Responsible Medical Officers (RMOs). It is anticipated that there will be three new roles:

- Approved Mental Health Professionals (AMHPs) (social work, mental health and learning disability nursing, clinical psychology or occupational therapy backgrounds)
- Approved Clinicians (ACs) (medicine, social work, mental health and learning disability nursing, clinical psychology or occupational therapy backgrounds)
- Responsible Clinicians (RCs) (medicine, social work, mental health and learning disability nursing, clinical psychology or occupational therapy backgrounds)

Mental health nurses may assume these roles once satisfactory training and governance arrangements are in place, and it is expected that training of AMHPs will have its base upon current ASW training, workforce modernisation and 'new ways of working'. In a similar way to nurse training, mental health work is an integral part of all social work education and practice experience, reflecting social work's commitment to an holistic approach to the individual in families and communities.

The Role of the Occupational Therapist

The number of occupational therapists registered to work across the health and social care sectors in the UK totals over 26,000. It is estimated that about 30% of these work in mental health (College of Occupational Therapy [COT], 2006).

Occupational therapists have developed an increasingly broad range of skills in the mental health arena, including assessment and advisory roles on the provision of aids and adaptations. They increasingly provide therapy programmes and specialist support and treatment to those with restricted activity levels or limited ability to participate as a result of their mental health issues. Their aim is to promote the highest level of independence possible.

A state registered occupational therapist (OT) works in partnership with the patient, carer, mental health nurses and other healthcare and voluntary personnel as part of the multidisciplinary team. OTs may be involved at all stages of mental health care, from acute episodes, through recovery, to outpatient and community and day care.

Occupational therapy is provided by both qualified and support staff and is concerned with the nature, balance, pattern and context of activities and occupations in the lives of the individual, their family and the community in which they exist. The aim of occupational therapy is to promote the clients' optimum potential, and supporting recovery, health, well-being and social participation.

This is achieved by the occupational therapist identifying the elements, which make up a person's ability to carry out selected activities (i.e. physical, cognitive, perceptual, psychological, social, environmental and spiritual), and will include jointly-agreed goals and activity. OTs use purposeful activity to promote rehabilitation and recovery through the restoration of function, hopefully maximising engagement in meaningful activities (i.e. occupations of self-care, domestic, social and work activity).

COT (2007) suggest that the more skilful the intervention the occupational therapist makes, the smaller the 'footprint' they leave, and postulate that success in this is demonstrated when service users feel that they have made the intervention themselves. This aspiration is very relevant to mental health nursing and other members of the MDT, and as with all accountable professionals it is important to be able to articulate and provide evidence of the basis of their therapeutic interventions and treatment at all levels.

The core skills of occupational therapy are defined by the COT and are built around occupation and activity. These include:

- Collaboration with the service user —building a collaborative relationship with the client that will promote reflection, autonomy and engagement in the therapeutic process
- Assessment — assessing and observing functional potential, limitations and needs including the effects of physical and psychosocial environments

- Enablement — enabling people to explore, achieve and maintain balance in the activities of daily living in the areas of personal care, domestic, leisure and productive activities
- Problem-solving — identifying and solving occupational performance problems
- Using activity as a therapeutic tool — using activities to promote health, well-being and function by analysing, devising, adapting, grading and applying activities for specific therapeutic purposes
- Group work — planning, organising and leading activity groups.

OT education is broad, covering mental and physical health, development, learning and the influence of context and culture in fulfilling occupations and as identified within the introduction increasingly inter professional in nature.

The Role of the Pharmacist

Traditionally the contact between pharmacists and people with mental health problems has been at the point of dispensing medication. However, pharmacists have more contact with the general public than any other health professional (Pharmaceutical Services Negotiating Committee [PSNC], 2003) and are therefore well placed to recognise early symptoms of mental health problems, identify signs of relapse, and help with concordance. This is particularly evident in primary care. This broad role of the pharmacist actively encourages good mental health practice, and can help to reduce stigma, helping change the public attitude towards mental health.

As with the other professions in the MDT, pharmacy is undergoing change to meet the demands of a modernised health service. *New Ways of Working* (DH, 2007) initiatives have identified pharmacy staff as a groups that can develop new roles. This can occur in three ways:

- Development of the roles of staff working within pharmacy to release the time of pharmacists and pharmacy technicians to develop improved services
- Development of the roles of pharmacy staff to release time of other mental healthcare professionals and improve services to users
- Development of other staff to undertake work related to the management of medicines.

This last element is of particular importance to mental health nurses who work closely with pharmacists to devise plans where the patient takes responsibility to self administer their medication as a part of their recovery plan. In this case the pharmacist develops a plan of education for the patient in conjunction with the MDT and usually facilitated by the mental health nurse. The patient will be given a range of relevant information about indications, contra-indications and side effects of their medication, how and when to take it and what to do if things go wrong. The patient will undergo a graded exposure to taking the responsibility for their self-administration and the pharmacist will oversee progress through regular MDT meetings and reviews. This process is unique to hospital pharmacy, however the use of dosset boxes and blister packs have been established for some time and are increasingly becoming incorporated into the supply of medicines from community pharmacists.

The benefits of hospital pharmacy work are described by *NHS Careers* (2007) and provide an insight into the extended roles contemporary pharmacists undertake which include, particularly, a direct involvement in patient care, influencing treatment choices by being involved in decision making at the point of prescribing.

The Pharmacist working in primary care may become involved in:

- Prescribing advice and support for GPs
- Advice and encouragement on medicines usage for users and carers within the pharmacy
- Working with local user groups and day centre services
- Training others involved in supporting users and carers about medicines issues (for example home carers)

However, for most community mental health teams, comprehensive medicine-related services have been considered beyond the ability of the local independent pharmacist, although pharmacists may well argue that they have recognised and responded to people with mental health needs, providing not only medication but advice for their customers to develop informed understanding of the medication they have been prescribed. High street pharmacists have extended their role in this respect, and consequently primary care has benefited from this development.

The Role of the Voluntary Sector

The voluntary sector consists of highly skilled professional organisations who work collaboratively to achieve high quality services for people with mental health problems. Government policy demands that patients are central to development of services, and the voluntary sector have a track record of innovative project work which can inform and assist development of quality services.

There are over half a million voluntary and community groups in the UK, ranging from small community groups to large national or international organisations. An increasing number of public services are delivered by voluntary and community organisations on behalf of the Government, and every area across the UK has independent local advocates who may be called upon to provide a 'voice' for patients in the context of multidisciplinary care.

In defining the voluntary sector, terms like 'charity sector', the 'not-for-profit sector' and the 'third sector' are often used interchangeably. At its broadest, the sector includes organisations registered with the Charity Commission, as well as a vast array of others, including housing associations, schools, places of worship, trade unions, sports and recreation clubs, and small voluntary groups.

As the sector continues to expand and there has been a significant growth in terms of roles and responsibilities. Some examples of national voluntary sector organisations that influence mental health are:

- The Mental Health Foundation (innovative research and practice)
- Mind — the National Association for Mental Health (federation of many local associations across England and Wales)
- Rethink — previously the National Schizophrenia Fellowship (particular interest in carers' issues)
- The Alzheimers Disease Society (research and support for those affected by dementia)
- Young Minds (mental health in children and young adults).

Locally, each NHS Trust has a Patient Advice and Liaison Service (PALS) to provide information, confidential advice and support to help patients, families and their carers. Their general aims are to provide an accessible gateway to information about the local NHS Trust and a 'one stop shop' for resolving any concerns about the organisation for patients, carers, or those who simply live in the local area.

The Private Sector

The private sector is profit making and provides a range of hospital and community-based mental health services. People using these services must pay for their own care or receive funding from elsewhere. In certain circumstances, health and social services may provide funding for care by an independent provider. The term 'independent healthcare' refers to any private, voluntary, not-for-profit or independent healthcare establishment under the regulatory remit of the Healthcare Commission. This is defined as any establishment (or service, agency, practice or business) required to register with the Commission under the Care Standards Act 2000, as amended by the Health and Social Care Act 2003, and also comply with Private and Voluntary Health Care (England) Regulations 2001.

Learning Points

1. The multidisciplinary team consists of a broad range of professional groups who collaborate their knowledge and expertise for the benefit of the service user.

References

Borrill C, West M, Dawson J, Shapiro D, Rees A, Richards A, Garrod S, Carletta J, Carter A (2000) Team Working and Effectivemess in Healthcare: Findings from the Health Care Team Effectiveness Project. *Br J Health Care Manage* **6:** 364–71

Carter S, Garside P, Black A (2003) Multidisciplinary team working, clinical networks, and chambers; opportunities to work differently in the NHS. *Qual Saf Health Care* **12:** 25–8

COT (2006) *Recovering Ordinary Lives: The strategy for occupational therapy in mental health services 2007–2017. A vision for the next ten years.* College of Occupational Therapists, London

CHI (2004) *Commission for Health Improvement. NHS National Staff Survey.* The Stationery Office, London

DH (1997) *The New NHS: Modern, Dependable.* The Stationery Office, London

DH (1998) *A First Class Service: Quality in the New NHS (White Paper).* The Stationery Office, London

Freeman M, Miller C, Ross N (2000) The impact of individual philosophies of teamwork on multiprofessional practice and its implications for education. *J Interprofessional Care* **14**(3): 40–4

HM Treasury (2004) V*oluntary And Community Sector Review 2004. Working Together, Better Together.* HM Treasury, London

Mohrman SA,Cohen SG, Mohrman AM Jr (1995) *Designing Team-Based Organisations.* Jossey-Bass, San Francisco

NHS Executive (1999) *Clinical Governance: Quality in the New NHS.* NHSE, London

PSNC (2003) *Pharmaceutical Services Negotiating Committee National Service Framework for Mental Health: A guide for community pharmacists.* PSNC, London

Schon DA (1983) *The Reflective Practitioner.* Jossey-Bass, San Francisco

Zaccaro S, Rittman A, Marks M (2001) Team leadership. *The Leadership Quaterly* **12**(4): 451–83

CHAPTER 4

The Role of the Psychiatrist Within the Multidisciplinary Team

Daniel Kinnair

The role of the consultant psychiatrist in the multidisciplinary setting is currently undergoing great changes. The Department of Health (DH) has set out in its document *New Ways of Working for Psychiatrists* (DH, 2005), a vision of how the consultant psychiatrist role might be in the future. Many of these changes aim to reduce individual case loads to enable consultants to work in a truly consultative fashion, and give priority to patients who have complex and severe disabilities. These changes to the role of the psychiatrist have been mirrored in the NHS by changes in the structure of teams, and the creation of new teams, such as home treatment and crisis resolution services. These new teams are often led by nurse and allied professionals, with a small number of psychiatrists assessing the severely disabled or high risk patients.

In this chapter I have used a traditional community mental health team in general adult psychiatry to illustrate the role of the psychiatrist within a multidisciplinary team. Psychiatrists working in community mental health teams may work in several different multidisciplinary teams. They may cover a geographic catchment area, and work within a community team.

The psychiatrist may also have a number of inpatient beds at a local psychiatric unit and work with a multidisciplinary team based there. The psychiatrist may also work with a local crisis team, home treatment team or assertive outreach team. The role of the psychiatrist within these teams may have subtle differences, but this chapter will explore in detail the extent of this role.

Training to be a Consultant Psychiatrist

Before considering in more detail the role of the psychiatrist within multidisciplinary teams, we should consider what training is required to qualify as a consultant psychiatrist. Psychiatrists, like GPs, surgeons, cardiologists, and other medical doctors have undertaken a common basic training at medical school. A medical degree in the UK takes between 4 to 6 years, depending on previous qualifications. Medical students study anatomy, physiology, sociology, psychology, pharmacology, and basic sciences, and also learn how to take a history from patients and perform physical examinations. This is in contrast to clinical psychologists, who have studied psychology, but not medicine. Medical students rotate between hospital and community specialities, and perhaps spend on average eight weeks in various psychiatric units, and attached to community mental health teams. At the end of the medical school, the students will hope to pass final exams to become junior doctors. At this point in their careers junior doctors need to begin to make some decisions about their career path.

In August 2005 the way in which junior doctors are trained in the UK changed through a process known as *Modernising Medical Careers* (DH, 2004). From August 2005 newly qualified doctors now spend two years as foundation year doctors. These foundation doctors rotate every four months between a choice of specialities, one of which may be in psychiatry. Towards the end of their foundation years the junior doctors have to apply for speciality training. If a doctor applies for psychiatry training they will then spend six years training to become a consultant psychiatrist. During these six years they must spend time in various psychiatric specialities and learn how to assess, diagnose, and treat patients with mental health problems. Junior doctors also observe the ways in which other professionals within the multidisciplinary team work, and develop the skills and knowledge to jointly work with staff both in the community and on inpatient units. During the first three years of this training the junior doctor must pass a number of examinations, both written and clinical, set by the Royal College of Psychiatrists (RCP). Passing these examinations allows individual junior doctors to become members of the College, and hence proceed with training.

During the last three years of training, following successful completion of the Royal college examinations, the doctor will choose to specialise in one specific field of psychiatry (for example general adult psychiatry), and learn how to take on the roles of a consultant psychiatrist.

The Multidisciplinary Team

Multidisciplinary team working, although still in its infancy in some areas of medicine, has been the mainstay of psychiatric services for many years. The needs of patients with severe and enduring mental health problems requires a multi-disciplinary approach, as no one professional group is equipped with all of the necessary skills, knowledge and attitudes to meet that need.

Working in teams can at times be difficult and the General Medical Council (GMC) has set out a series of points which they consider to be essential to good medical practice when working in teams (GMC, 2006). These include:

- Respect the skills and contributions of your colleagues
- Maintain professional relationships with patients
- Communicate effectively with colleagues within and outside the team
- Make sure that your patients and colleagues understand your professional status and speciality, your role and responsibilities in the team and who is responsible for each aspect of patients' care
- Participate in regular reviews and audit of the standards and performance of the team, taking steps to remedy any deficiencies
- Be willing to deal openly and supportively with problems in the performance, conduct or health of team members.

Over the last 30 years there has been a drive nationally to close psychiatric asylums and move towards community mental health teams. In many parts of the UK there are multidisciplinary teams, which include psychiatrists, psychologists, nurses, occupational therapists, social workers, physiotherapists, speech therapists, pharmacists and voluntary service workers, and these teams treat individuals as in-patients, day patients and outpatients. By the early 1990s over 85% of England and Wales was covered by a sector community mental health team, (Johnson and Thornicroft, 1993). More recently this drive has seen the introduction of more than 700 specialised multi-disciplinary mental health teams, including 252 assertive outreach teams, 343 crisis resolution teams, and 118 early intervention teams (Appleby, 2007). The Mental Health Act of 1959 first established in law the necessary relationship between the health service (psychiatrists and nurses), and social services (social workers). This relationship has continued, and within the Trust in which I work this is a formal partnership between health and social services.

In a Royal College of Psychiatrists publication, (Community Mental Health Care, 2005), three distinct functions of a generic community mental health team are described:

- Assessment and advice on management for patients treated in primary care by general practitioners

- Providing treatment and care for time limited disorders which are more complex or severe than those treatable in primary care
- Providing treatment and care for those with severe and enduring needs.

We will now continue to examine the role of the consultant psychiatrist within a generic community mental health team.

Role of the Psychiatrist within the MDT

A consultant in general adult psychiatry has been defined as 'a specialist in the diagnosis and assessment, management and prevention of the full range of mental health disorders affecting adults of working age' (RCP, 2006).

Within a generic community mental health team there may be one consultant psychiatrist, who is in turn responsible for several junior trainee psychiatrists. The consultant may run outpatient clinics, do home visits, and also have in-patients at a local psychiatric unit. The consultant may also have a role working out of normal office hours, assessing emergency referrals, and may have input into home treatment, and crisis resolution services. However, importantly the consultant should also attend team meetings where new referrals are discussed, difficult cases reviewed, and team supervision and support given. The psychiatrist is not usually the team manager, but they have a key role in the team.

Specific Roles of the Psychiatrist

The following description of the specific roles of the psychiatrist is based on the guidance given by the Royal College of Psychiatrists (RCP, 2006).

Assessment

Referrals are made to community mental health teams by GPs, primary care workers/therapists, other hospital-based specialists, and between community teams as patients move between sectors. GPs expect between 70 and 80% of assessments of new patients to be by trained psychiatrists, either singly or jointly with other disciplines (RCP, 2005). New referrals are often discussed in a weekly team meeting, where all members of the multidisciplinary team are present. The referrals to the team will then be allocated to appropriate team members, depending on the nature of the referral. Consultant psychiatrists have the option of reviewing the patient in an outpatient clinic, or if the case is urgent or there is a risk of non-attendance, organising to see the patient at home. However, in

---

CASE 2.1

A referral is made to a Community Mental Health Team (CMHT) by a GP. The patient, Mr Smith, has presented to the GP with a fear of dirt and contamination. Due to this fear the patient is repeatedly washing his hands and has found it difficult to go to work. This problem has been getting worse now for two months and the GP believes the patient has an obsessive compulsive disorder (OCD), and wonders if cognitive behavioural therapy (CBT) will help. The GP has started the patient on an antidepressant which is licensed for use in OCD.

The referral is discussed at the CMHT weekly meeting and it is agreed that it could be a case of OCD. One of the Community Psychiatric Nurses (CPN), has trained in CBT for OCD, and the case is allocated to the CPN, Liz, to assess and treat the patient. It is agreed that Liz should feedback the progress to the team in the meeting in one months time.

Liz sees Mr Smith at home, and is struck by how depressed he is. Liz does not feel that CBT is appropriate and speaks to the psychiatrist within the team, who agrees to see Mr Smith for an assessment.

---

many cases the referral will be allocated to another member of the team if that is appropriate. An example of this is highlighted in *Case 2.1*.

Psychiatrists are trained to understand and weigh in the balance developmental, biological, social and psychological factors in the presentation of mental disease, and arise at a diagnostic appraisal taking into account relevant cultural factors. When assessing a new patient a psychiatrist would take a full history of the presenting complaint, undertake a social and personal history, and perform a mental state examination. The history would also include a consideration of substance misuse, forensic issues, and a medical history. This would enable a diagnostic formulation to be made and a treatment plan could then be discussed and agreed with the patient. Throughout the history the psychiatrist will also formulate a thorough risk assessment.

A medically qualified psychiatrist is not the only individual with the necessary training and experience to complete an assessment and reach a diagnosis. Experienced community nurses, occupational therapists, psychologists, and primary care workers also develop skills in recognising key features of psychiatric illness, and can make accurate diagnosis. However, when the presentation is complicated or there is uncertainty, a team member may ask for an opinion from the psychiatrist as to the diagnosis. This is often important if a patient has been known to a team member for a long period of time and there appears to have been no progress in treatment, or if there has been a change in the patients' presentation.

Treatment

Treatment plans need to be drawn up with the patient, and a bio-psychosocial approach is often considered. Having reached a diagnosis during the assessment, the consultant psychiatrist can use this information to offer the most appropriate and up-to-date treatment available. It is therefore imperative that a psychiatrist keeps up-to-date with recent research surrounding treatment and diagnostic issues.

Depending on the diagnosis, treatment may involve a pharmacological approach (medication), a psychological approach (a psychological therapy, such as cognitive behavioural therapy), or a social approach (day care, home care, or planned activities).

Within the team many of the decisions regarding medication are taken either by, or in discussion with, the psychiatrist as he or she would be the only medically qualified team member. However, recently with the introduction of nurse prescribing courses some of the prescribing role no longer requires a psychiatrist, except for more complicated cases. Many psychiatrists are familiar with, and may be trained in a variety of psychological therapies, such as CBT, or psychodynamic psychotherapy. However, given the length and time commitment needed by the therapist, the psychiatrist may not be able to undertake this type of work routinely. Specific members of the CMHT may have specific and specialised knowledge about psychological therapies, and after the assessment, the psychiatrist may refer the patient to another member of the team for treatment. Treatment may involve liaison with many different specialities, and with the voluntary sector and with families and carers to maximise treatment efficacy.

All patients seen by mental health teams are required to be on the care programme approach (DH, 1990). As part of care programme approach there is often a need for a multi-disciplinary review, when all members of the community team, appropriate voluntary agencies, families, carers, the individual, and if required an advocate, should be present to review treatment and progress. See *Case 2.2* below for an example.

The Mental Health Act 1983

The Mental Health Act of 1983 sets out in law the roles and responsibilities of psychiatrists, nurses and approved social workers. In practice the act allows patients suffering with a severe mental illness, where there is an associated element of risk, either to health, or the patients' safety through suicide, or risk to others, to be detained in a place of safety, (for example, a hospital), and to receive treatment.

I have highlighted how the psychiatrist must engage with other professions to use the mental health act in *Case 2.3*.

CASE 2.2

The psychaitrist, Dr Jones, assesses Mr Smith — the patient from Case 2.1 at the request of Liz, the CPN. It is clear from the history that Mr Smith has an OCD, but he is also suffering from a severe depressive episode, although there are no current suicidal thoughts. At the end of the interview Dr Jones, Mr Smith, Mr Smiths' wife, and Liz, discuss the treatment plan.

Dr Jones agrees to change Mr Smiths' antidepressant, and gives him a new prescription. Dr Jones organises to see Mr. Smith in six weeks to assess his progress on this new antidepressant, and if necessary make further changes.

In the meantime, Liz will visit once a fortnight to assess and monitor Mr Smith's mood, and will feedback to Dr Jones if there are any concerns. Liz will not start the CBT for OCD until Mr Smith's mood has lifted. Mr and Mrs Smith are given contact numbers for the team, and an emergency telephone number for out of hours problems.

Dr Jones agrees to sign a sickness certificate for the next six weeks until he reviews Mr Smith in clinic again.

Teaching and Audit

With a wealth of knowledge and experience, a consultant psychiatrist is ideally placed to take on a lead role in teaching and educational activities. Sadly, in many centres teaching and educational activities are often not multidisciplinary in nature and are instead aimed at single groups of staff. All members of the multidisciplinary team have specialised skills and knowledge in their field, and this can be shared at educational events, which can be included in weekly team meetings.

Many psychiatrists are also involved in the teaching of students from a variety of disciplines, such as medical, nursing, and psychology undergraduates. Consultant psychiatrists often have junior trainee psychiatrists working with them. The consultant has a role as trainer and educational supervisor for these junior doctors. Consultants themselves are also now engaging in a process of continual professional development,

CASE 2.3

During one of her visits to see Mr Smith, Liz notices that he seems increasingly low in mood despite the change in medication. Mr Smith confides that he feels desperate and has been stockpiling paracetamol, as he feels that life is not worth living. He plans to take a large overdose when his wife goes out to work. Liz immediately contacts Dr Jones and they agree that Mr Smith will need an in-patient admission until his medication is optimised.

Liz discusses this with Mr Smith, but he states that he does not want to go to hospital as he cannot see how it can help. He states he can see no way out and wishes to die. Liz contacts Dr Jones again and a decision is taken to organise a Mental Health Act assessment at Mr Smith's house. Liz agrees to stay with Mr Smith until the team arrive.

Dr Jones speaks to Mr Smith's GP, Dr Shah, and they agree to meet at Mr Smith's house. Dr Jones also contacts Sue Douglas, an approved social worker, who also agrees to attend.

The two doctors and social worker talk to Mr Smith. He is clearly severely depressed and the team agree he is at high risk of suicide. The team try to persuade Mr Smith to come to hospital, but he refuses. The doctors complete independent medical recommendations for a Section 3 of the Mental Health Act. The social worker completes the section. Mr Smith has been detained under Section 3, and can now be transferred to the local psychiatric unit for treatment of his depressive illness.

On arrival Mr Smith is seen by a junior doctor working with Dr Jones and Brian, one of the ward nurses, and is formally admitted to hospital.

and are themselves classed as learners, with ongoing educational needs. To continue to practice consultants need to attend a number of hours of educational activities every year, and have a regular review with a peer. This process is to ensure that consultants stay up to date with developments in the field of mental health, and can offer patients an evidence based approach to assessment and treatment.

Audit has been defined by NICE (2002) as:

'Clinical audit is a quality improvement process that seeks to improve patient care and outcomes through systematic review of care against explicit criteria and the implementation of change. Aspects of the structure, processes, and outcomes of care are selected and systematically evaluated

against explicit criteria. Where indicated changes are implemented at an individual, team, or service level, and further monitoring is used to confirm improvement in healthcare delivery.'

NICE, 2002

In the example cases included in this chapter there are several obvious criteria that might be examined in an audit. These are:

- How long did Mr Smith have to wait to be seen by the team? (waiting times are often set to a maximum number of weeks.)
- When treating Mr. Smiths' depression did Dr. Jones follow NICE (2004) guidelines on depression?
- Was the Mental Health Act paperwork filled out correctly?
- During the admission to the ward, was Mr. Smith clerked in fully by the nurse and junior doctor, using the locally approved process set out by the hospital?

As a consultant psychiatrist we can encourage audit activities within the team, institute changes in practice if necessary, and encourage a re-audit of practice to ensure standards of care are being achieved.

Clinical Supervision

A consultant psychiatrist may be responsible for the direct supervision of several junior trainee psychiatrists within the team. Many psychiatrists also provide clinical supervision for other team members especially with difficult and complex cases.

Leadership and Management

Consultant psychiatrists are rarely team managers. The consultant is likely to only be the line manager for junior doctors working with him or her. However, as highly trained individuals consultants are expected to provide leadership in their clinical setting. Within community mental health teams, consultants may take on a leadership role to inspire and motivate the team, and by providing a clear vision of where the team is headed. At the present time in the NHS there is a great deal of change in the ways in which teams work, and this produces a great deal of anxiety in individuals and within teams. The role of an effective leader is to try to contain that anxiety, be an advocate for the team within the trust or foundation hospital, and provide a clear line of communication. Consultants are rarely the only leaders within teams, and there is an expectation that all senior staff will take on a leadership role. Depending on the task at hand the role of leader may alternate between team members.

Responsibilities of the Consultant Psychiatrist

At the present time there is much debate as to the nature and degree of responsibility carried by consultants with respect to patients being seen by them, by junior doctors working with them, and by members of the community mental health team. Consultants do not and should not be expected to know every patient open to the team. There has been an assumption previously that even if the consultant is only involved in the periphery of a patients care, they hold overall responsibility, and therefore are accountable.

Several modes of clinical responsibility were set out in the document, *Roles and Responsibilities of the Consultant in General Adult Psychiatry* (RCP, 2006), and these are:

- Direct responsibility — arises from direct clinical involvement in the case. For example patients seen only in outpatient clinics where no other team member is involved

---

Learning Points

1. Consultant psychiatrists are medically qualified doctors
2. It takes a minimum of 6 years training in psychiatry, and a set of post graduate qualifications to qualify as a consultant.
3. A consultant in general adult psychiatry has been defined as 'a specialist in the diagnosis and assessment, management and prevention of the full range of mental health disorders affecting adults of working age'
4. The needs of patients with severe and enduring mental health problems requires a multi-disciplinary approach, as no one professional group is equipped with all of the necessary skills, knowledge and attitudes to meet that need.
5. Consultant psychiatrists have a number of roles within a team, but have a central role with patients detained under the mental health act 1983.
6. Consultant psychiatrists may be engaged in audit, teaching and research.
7. The ways in which consultant psychiatrists work is currently changing in many parts of the country.
8. Responsibility for patient care can be divided into direct, delegated and distributed responsibility within multidisciplinary teams.

- Delegated responsibility — the consultant delegates some or all aspects of care to other professionals. Every professional within the community mental health team however, is responsible for the quality of care they provide
- Distributed responsibility — responsibility for the care of the individual is distributed amongst the professionals involved, according to their role and contribution. The case example in this chapter sets out a situation where Dr Jones and Liz the community psychiatric nurse distribute responsibility whilst providing care, treatment, monitoring and support in the community.

References

Appleby L (2007) *Breaking Down Barriers Clinical Case for Change.* DH, London

DH (2005) *New Ways of Working for Psychiatrists: Enhancing effective person centred services through new ways of working in multidisciplinary and multiagency contexts. Final report 'but not the end of the story'.* DH, London

DH (2004) *Modernising Medical Careers: The next steps.* DH, London

DH (1990) *The Care Programme Approach for People with a Mental Illness Referred to the Psychiatric Services.* Joint Health/Social Services Circular HC (90) 23/LASS (90)11. DH, London

GMC (2006) *Good Medical Practice.* GMC, LOndon

Johnson S, Thornicroft G (1993) The sectorisation of psychiatry services in England and Wales. *Soc Psychiatr Psychiatric Epidemiol* **28**: 45–7

NICE (2002) *Principles for Best Practice in Clinical Audit.* NICE, London

NICE (2004) *Depression: Management of Depression in Primary and Secondary Care.* National Clinical Practice Guideline number 23. NICE, London

RCP (2006) *Roles and Responsibilities of the Consultant in General Adult Psychiatry.* Royal College of Psychiatrists, London

RCP (2005) *Community Mental Health Care.* Royal College of Psychiatrists, London

CHAPTER 5

The Role of the Psychologist Within the Multidisciplinary Team

Sally Rudge

Psychologists work in a wide variety of health care settings, from in-patient to community based, working with all age groups either individually, as couples, families, groups, organisations or communities. They work with people of all abilities including learning disabilities and brain injury, those experiencing mental health problems, and a range of physical health problems.

The majority of psychologists working within health and social care settings are clinical psychologists, although there are a growing number of other psychologists increasingly represented in the multidisciplinary team (MDT). Counselling psychologists have lifted the expectations and efficacy of counselling, and together with their colleagues in forensic, health and occupational psychology are further enhancing the depth and breadth of the MDT. This chapter will focus on the general roles of psychologists working in contemporary mental heath care rather than discuss the differences between these groups as there are many common competences and expectations when working within an MDT.

The underpinning philosophy of psychologists, and one that is based upon the core purpose and philosophy of the profession is:

'...based on the fundamental acknowledgement that all people have the same human value, and the right to be treated as unique individuals. Clinical psychologists will treat all people — both clients and colleagues — with dignity and respect and will work with them collaboratively as equal partners towards the achievement of mutually agreed goals.'

Harvey, 2001

The purpose of the profession is to reduce psychological distress and to enhance and promote psychological well-being by the systematic application of knowledge derived from psychological theory and data (Harvey, 2001)

On an individual level, clinical psychologists aim to enable and equip individuals with the necessary skills and knowledge to manage their daily lives in such a way that they are achieving their optimal level of psychological and physical wellbeing and, like mental health nurses, the importance of the therapeutic relationship is paramount. This includes:

- Enabling the client/patient to become hopeful about their circumstances
- Encouraging the client/patient to recognise their own personal responsibilities in the resolution of their issues
- Providing learning opportunities for the client/patient to enable self reflection and to acknowledge progress and achievement
- Encouraging the client/patient to self-advocate
- Promoting the clients ability to develop and maintain support systems which enhance their abilities and coping strategies.

In order to achieve these aims, the psychologist uses a set of core skills: assessment, formulation, intervention and evaluation.

This assessment is different from those carried out by other members of the MDT in that psychologists have a number of specific psychometric and psychological tests available for them to use. Testing the client/patient mood, personality, intelligence, social functioning and neuropsychological function may be seen as central to the psychologists' role. Mental health nurses are able to carry out some of the tests traditionally reserved for psychologists following post-registration training. Some elements of assessment are common with other MDT professionals, and include interviewing, observation, and devising self-monitoring strategies. The nursing process in mental health nursing considers four elements:

- Assessment
- Planning
- Implementation
- Evaluation.

In psychology, the focus is on assessment, formulation and evaluation. There are very clear parallels between these two frameworks and both are compatible in the keeping of multidisciplinary notes.

The assessment process considers the psychological processes and behaviour of an individual, and seeks to gain an awareness of change and stability which has happened for the individual, and also to compare them with others.

Formulation is the summation and integration of the knowledge that is acquired by the assessment process (Harvey, 2001). The aim of a formulation is to gain a psychological understanding of the problem, how it developed, and how it is being maintained.

Using a range of psychological models and theories the information gained from the assessment is reviewed, evaluated, analysed, and provisional hypotheses are produced. From the formulation any intervention plans, if required, can be devised.

Evaluation both whilst interventions are ongoing, and when it comes to an end, are used to assess the stability and security of change.

What Psychologists bring to the MDT

In the same way as the nursing and medical profession have a national governing body, psychology has the British Psychological Society (BPS), which is the representative body for psychology and psychologists in the UK, and the only body in the UK which covers all areas of psychology. It monitors the quality of its members and their professional practice. It sets standards, and promotes the quality of psychological interventions for service users.

Whilst it is acknowledged that there are other members of an MDT, particularly the mental health nurse, who can use competently a variety of psychological interventions, the psychologist is the team member whose sole focus is on psychological processes and behaviour of the clients. The psychologist is therefore the psychological intervention expert member of the MDT, by virtue of the training undertaken.

The psychological formulation is complementary to the other assessments completed by other MDT professionals, including the psychiatric diagnosis, and broadens the understanding of the problems presented, thus aiding in producing an effective plan for intervention.

Psychologists not only bring their skills as psychological therapists to an MDT, as a scientist-practitioner they also have a role in ongoing research to increase the pool of theory-based knowledge which in turn allows for an increase in evidence-based practice.

The *Guidelines for Clinical Psychology Services* (BPS, 2004) aim to ensure that the skills and expertise of the psychologist are used to give the most effect. A section of the guidelines address the role of the psychologist with the MDT, and calls for very clear definition of duties and expectations.

As psychological interventions are delivered by other professionals, and with the length and depth of training received, it is expected that psychologists will be a resource for MDT staff, and share and develop the psychological knowledge and skills of all MDT workers.

This not only suggests that the psychologist uses their research skills for complex audit and evaluation, and develop their own evidence-based practice through research, but that there is a sharing of information with the MDT, and collaborative working to produce evidence-based practice or research-based initiatives and service evaluation which will enhance and develop the service given by the team to the client.

With their knowledge of group processes, the psychological perspective is a positive attribute to effective team working. *Working in Teams* (BPS, 2001) recognises that effective psychologists are not isolated from the other disciplines that provide healthcare, and places the role of psychology firmly within the MDT. The psychologist is well placed to support the team with their own psychological needs. This may include facilitating peer support, or taking part in the clinical supervision of other team members.

There is, however, some degree of difficulty in being fully embraced by the MDT, in that although the contribution of psychology is welcomed, the proximity and access to psychologists may be problematic. Psychology services have traditionally operated within office hours and this has limited the integration of psychology into the team. The *Best Practice Guidelines* issued by the BPS suggest that a psychologist is the sole or majority user of their office (BPS, 2004). A single office enables the psychologist to work effectively in terms of confidential conversations and an environment that is conducive to therapeutic engagement, but it may be unhelpful in developing and maintaining good MDT relations. On the otehr hand, shared office space with other disciplines prevents professional isolation, and promotes inter-professional collaboration.

The Future of the Psychologist in the MDT

As with other professions within the MDT, the psychology service is adapting to meet the needs of the service user. These factors have been addressed with a number of service reviews in both NHS and private sector psychology services.

The *Layard Report* (Layard, 2004) suggested that people with mental health problems should have easy access to psychological therapies, in particular to cognitive behavioural therapy, as the recommended approach to the most common mental health problems (DH, 2007). It was argued that a shortage of psychologists caused waiting lists to rise. The *Layard Report* promoted increasing the number of psychologists, and recommended a change in the way psychologists are used. It suggested that psychologists have a supervisory and consultative role which is more managerial in nature. They would be the hub of a 'hub and spoke' model of care with nurses, occupational therapists and social workers who have had training in CBT, delivering the majority of the therapy. Graduate mental health workers and associate psychologists would also have a role in the stepped care approach to achieving access to all who would benefit from psychological therapies.

The Government in 2005 made a manifesto commitment to increase access to psychological therapies for the people who needed help from mental health services.

New Ways of Working for Applied Psychologists (Lavender and Hope, 2006) is an ongoing project which aims to address seven objects which include identifying the best ways that applied psychologists can contribute to the development and work of multidisciplinary teams.

Improving Access to Psychological Therapies (DH, 2007) aims to deliver the Government's 2005 manifesto commitment to provide access to psychological therapies for people with mental health problems. Using pilot demonstration sites and eight Regional Development Centres, the aim has been to develop and assess the effectiveness in practice of some of the recommendations put forward.

Throughout all of the changes that will be taking place in the future, it is clear that there will be a role for a growing team of applied psychologists and associates within the MDT.

The British Psychological Society has identified the unique contribution psychology makes to mental health work, and it is adopting a multi professional perspective and taking into account the implications and reviews of other professional groups which are considering *New Ways of Working* (for example *New Ways of Working for Psychiatrists* [Royal College of Psychiatrists, 2005]; *Social Workers* [CSIP, 2006]; *Mental Health Nursing Review* [DH, 2006]; *Allied Health Professionals* [CSIP and NIMHE, 2007]).

There are a number of core professional activities for psychologists delivering therapeutic services. The BPS suggest that psychologists are essentially problem-solvers, formulating problems and questions in psychological terms and drawing creatively on a wealth of psychological theories and techniques from the discipline of psychology to find ways forward. These include:

- Assessment, whereby the psychologist seeks to gain an understanding of the difficulties from the client perspective, taking into account the wider context
- Formulation to develop with the client(s) a psychological explanation of how and why the particular difficulties have arisen and are experienced by the client(s)
- Planning and implementation of a course of psychological therapy

- Evaluation of the outcome of the therapy
- Management of services in the NHS, public and private sectors
- Supervision and training of other counselling psychologists, applied psychologists, assistant psychologists and other related professionals
- Multidisciplinary team work and team facilitation
- Service and organisational development, leadership and management (policy development/change management)
- Audit and evaluation
- Research and development

The unique contribution made by psychologists is, in part, counterbalanced by the development of inter-professional learning and education, whereby nurses, psychologists, social workers and medics come together with colleagues from audiology and in some cases occupational therapy to learn some of the overlapping principles that govern health work. Psychology differs from nursing in that it is an all-graduate profession, while mental health nursing still has a diploma entry route.

It is anticipated that the psychology training of the future will remain graduate-based with a career framework for these graduates through to doctorate level training. This will mean the creation of at least two levels of pre-qualification post, namely that of Psychology Assistant and Psychology Associate. A model supported by Lavender and Hope (2006) sets out the career development for a career in psychology (See *Figure 3.1*).

Within the new career frameworks, it is proposed that qualified mental health nurses and other professionals who demonstrate specialist competence

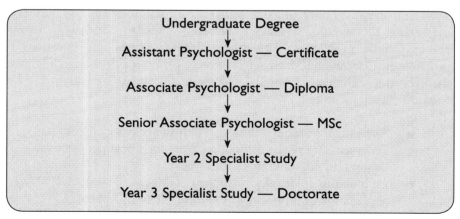

Figure 3.1 Proposed model for career development in psychology (Lavender and Hope, 2006)

in psychological therapies will be able to become psychological therapists, and non-chartered applied psychologists delivering psychological therapies, who will be regulated with registration. It is anticipated that the therapists will work at an equivalent level to the assistant or associate psychologist depending on experience and academic pathway. The route for different divisions within the profession is also converging with the potential for clinical, health and counselling sharing academic and clinical progress together within this model.

Learning Points

1. Psychologists work as specialists in the MDT and their methods are compatible with those that mental health nurses use
2. People with mental health problems should have easy access to psychological therapies, in particular to cognitive behavioural therapy, as the recommended approach to the most common mental health problems
3. The user's perspectives and experience are critically important to the role
4. The role of the psychologist is expanding, and the opportunities for mental health nurses to shape their career within the field of psychology is being actively encouraged.

References

BPS (1998) *Guidelines for Clinical Psychology Services*. Division of Clinical Psychology, The British Psychological Society, Leicester

BPS (2001) *Working in Teams*. A report by the division of Clinical Psychology. The British Psychological Society, Leicester

CSIP (2006) *The Social Work Contribution to Mental Health Services. The Future Direction*. Report Of Responses to the Discussion Paper 21st March 2006. CSIP, London

CSIP, NIMHE (2007) *Mental Health: New Ways of Working for Everyone*. Developing and sustaining a capable and flexible workforce. CSIP and NIMHE, London

DH (2006) *Recruitment and Retention of Mental Health Nurses: Good Practice Guide*. DH, London

DH (2007) *Improving Access to Psychological Therapies (IAPT) Programme: Computerised cognitive behavioural therapy (cCBT) implementation guidance*. DH, London

Harvey P (2001) *The Core Purpose and Philosophy of the Profession*. BPS, Leicester

Lavender T, Hope R (2006) *New Ways of Working for Applied Psychologists*. Progress Report November. BPS, Leicester

Layard R (2004) *Mental Health: Britain's biggest social problem?* The Centre for Economic Performance, London School of Economics, London

RCP (2005) *New Ways of Working for Psychiatry*. Royal College of Psychiatrists, London

CHAPTER 6

The Therapeutic Relationship in Acute Settings

Barbara Monk Steel

There have been many changes in the delivery of mental health services over the last decade, and this has impacted on modern acute care settings. The role of the mental health nurse has been impacted by the need for nurses to extend their roles and take on tasks more traditionally seen as the role of the doctor (DH, 1999). Traditionally, mental health nurses have seen the therapeutic relationship as the cornerstone of their practice (Higgins et al, 2000) although the science of psychiatry and the medical model of treatment have used a more biological explanation of mental health and a different focus for nurses. (Gournay, 1996).

There is a contrast between biological approaches that emphasise physical treatment and containment, and humanistic models that emphasise choice, empowerment and consider the personal meaning of patient's experience (Johnstone, 2000; Barker, 2002).

Nurses within acute settings have the difficult task of integrating these approaches. There is a need for effective containment, risk assessment, and biological treatments. The therapeutic relationship is central to the nurse's role in patient care, and poor relationships will affect the patient's experience of their in-patient stay (DH, 2006a).

The priorities of the mental health nurse in acute settings are to:

- Develop a therapeutic relationship
- Maintain the safety of patients
- Help the patient and care team develop mutual goals for care and treatment
- Support the patient in working towards their own improved mental health.

Developing the Therapeutic Relationship

Communication and relationship-building skills are key tools of the acute mental health nurse (Barker, 1998; Freshwater, 2003; Mallett and Dougherty, 2000).

Research into mental health nursing in acute settings conducted by Higgins et al (1999) found that the success of the nurses relationship was dependant on a range of psychotherapeutic and interpersonal tasks, including:

- Displaying empathy
- Valuing patients as individuals
- Being a good listener
- Being a good communicator
- Providing emotional support
- Being available for patients.

The skills the nurse uses to do this are often interlinked. Valuing patients as individuals is the basis for the nurses's therapeutic relationship. This means the nurse must respect for the patient regardless of their behaviour. This involves giving the person time, respecting their wishes and treating them as an equal human being, if not an equal in power and knowledge. Time specifically given to engaging in therapeutic relationships and activities are crucial in busy acute inpatient settings (DH, 2006a). Giving attention to the patient involves focusing specifically on the messages being communicated by the patient and help gain a full and accurate understanding of the patient's experience. The nurse should use both non-verbal and verbal skills in order to communicate, including:

- Appropriate eye contact
- Open gestures
- Responsive tone of voice
- Responsive facial expression
- Appropriate proximity
- Consistency between verbal and nonverbal messages
- Reflecting factual and emotional content back to the patient
- Paraphrasing and summarising factual and emotional content
- Checking for understanding
- Using non judgemental language.

Being available for patients and spending time with them helps to communicate to the patient that the nurse values them as a person and conveys interest and concern.

Empathy is the ability to understand the other person's experience, however different that may be from the nurse's experience. This understanding makes links between the way the patient experiences themselves and others, and the person's emotional response to these experiences. This is a particularly skilled task in acute mental health settings, as the nature of the patient's experience is often affected by their mental state. The nurse has to develop the capacity to appreciate what life is like for that patient, with their specific delusions, hallucinations, social and personal situation. To be empathic the nurse needs to be self-aware, understand their own emotional states, be able to describe these states and recognise the behavioural cues for emotional states in others. The quality of being a good listener helps the nurse to go beyond the range of their own experience and begin to develop an appreciation of a patient's internal world. As the nurse develops experience at listening they may be able to use both their own experience and that of other patients they have known in order to create a tentative hypothesis about a patient's unique experience (Freshwater, 2003; Stickley and Freshwater, 2006; Watkins, 2001). In order for empathy to impact on the therapeutic relationship, the patient needs to experience the nurse as empathic. The nurse needs to be able to communicate their understanding in language that the patient is familiar with (Nelson-Jones, 2000; Reynolds and Scott, 2000).

Providing emotional support consists of allowing the patient time to experience and express their feelings, and helping the patient respond in a productive way to their feelings.

Being a good communicator involves all these skills, and also being able to focus non-verbal and verbal responses to help the patient to understand and manage their experience. The nurse will use all the verbal and non- verbal skills already discussed and add skills of information-giving and explanation.

The nurse in acute mental health settings will need to adjust the way they give information and respond to the patient depending on the patient's ability to concentrate and remember information. The inpatient population in this setting is largely made up of people with serious mental illness which has affected their capacity to care for themselves (DH, 1999; Cleary et al, 2005; Sainsbury Centre for Mental Health, 2005). The nurse needs to assess how the patient's current (and changing) mental state is affecting their capacity to process information and respond to others. This will involve observation of the following verbal and non-verbal aspects of communication from the patient:

- Facial expressions
- Personal space
- Body posture
- Gestures
- Voice tone and pitch
- Eye contact and direction of gaze
- Length and complexity of sentences
- Amount of information
- Pace of speech.

The nurse will also need to adjust these aspects of their own communication to respond effectively to the patient's communication style.

Reasons for Admissions

The development of Crisis Resolution Home Service Teams have created options and alternatives for treatment and support in order to reduce the need for admission to hospital in an acute mental health crisis. There needs to be a clear purpose for admission in order to facilitate appropriate care. This may be to:

- Promote self-care
- Provide a place of safety for patients
- Provide respite for carers
- Manage symptoms of mental disorders
- Manage risk to self or others.

Patients may be admitted suffering from a range of mental disorders, although the most common psychiatric diagnoses are mood disorder (depression more frequently than mania) and anxiety, schizophrenia and related psychosis (Thompson et al,2004; Sainsbury Centre for Mental Health, 1998).

The patient will experience a range of problems influenced by their mental state and the nurse needs to formulate a care plan based on the following principles:

- Maintaining safety
- Maintaining physical health and well being
- Developing a therapeutic relationship
- Managing medication regimes
- Managing/improving the patients mental state.

The admission process is an opportunity for engagement with the patient and the beginning of the assessment — the evaluation cycle.

The nurse's role on admission has two aspects, one is to welcome the patient to their new environment and help them adjust to the setting. The other aspect is to start the process of gathering information and implementing care.

Welcoming the patient involves giving information about the clinical area, showing the patient important places and help them become comfortable. This will include where they will be sleeping, where they can spend time, where they can obtain drinks, and where the toilets and washing facilities are located. It also involves introducing the patient to key people, for example the nurse conducting the admission process, and members of the team of nurses who will be taking care of the patient. Information about what is going to happen during and after the admission process should also be given, including information about the patient's rights.

The nurse needs to use a range of communication skills to do this, including writing down the information the patient needs. These skills need to take account of the patient's mental state and the normal anxiety which will be experienced during the admission process.

Assessment

Through the assessment process the nurse begins to gather the information needed to identify needs and problems formulate goals in collaboration with the patient, and develop the therapeutic relationship (DH, 2006b). What do nurses need to assess? This usually falls into the following categories:

- Symptoms
- Functioning (biological, psychological and emotional, social)
- Risk.

Assessment can be broad-based, aimed at gathering a wide range of information that can later be evaluated for significance, or specific focused assessment aimed at eliciting specific, targeted information. Broad-based assessment is interested in all areas of functioning, while specific assessment is designed to elicit detailed information that the nurse knows is needed.

Methods of assessment are both formal and informal, and interviewing is a formal method that makes use of relationship and interpersonal processes. Communication skills are central to this information-gathering process, and the nurse needs to use these skills selectively depending on the goal of their assessment.

Informal Interviewing

For broad-based assessments, skills of reflection and open questions are needed to invite the patient to expand on their experience, and what is significant to them.

In focused assessment the skills of paraphrasing and summarising can guide the patient to expand on specific areas which the nurse needs to explore, followed by closed questions to elicit very specific pieces of information. Closed questions help to elicit factual and concrete information and ensure accurate understanding. Closed questions can be: what; when; where; who; how; why.

Empathic statements may help the nurse to develop and deepen a relationship with the patient, leading to a greater trust and willingness to share experiences.

Through the interview the nurse can gain insight into the patients world, and assess the compatibility of the patient's understanding of their problems, aims and goals with the understanding, aims and goals of the mental health professionals caring for them. Interviewing the patient can give the nurse a wealth of information, some of which will be confirmed or supplemented or adjusted through observation.

During the initial interview the nurse will have gained insight into the patients' views of their problems and illness, the reasons they think they have been admitted, how well they are functioning physically, psychologically and socially, and their level of risk.

The nurse needs to take an external perspective and combine information from the patient's self reports with observation of how the patient is functioning. The principle foci of observation are the patient's:

- Behaviour
- Thoughts
- Physical symptoms
- Social interactions.

The nurse will develop baseline observations of significant areas of interest on admission, identifying frequency, duration and intensity of the behaviours, thoughts, physical experiences and social interaction observed.

These specific observations can then act as a benchmark to note improvement or deterioration in the patient, and measure the effectiveness of any interventions designed to improve the patient's health and functioning.

When making observations, it is important to record only what is observed and has occurred, and avoid attributing values and meaning. Mistakes can be made when inferring motivation and meaning from behaviour alone, and conclusions drawn need to be checked out against other evidence, including the patient's views and interpretation.

Formal Interviewing

Formal techniques for assessment include measurement tools such as checklists, questionnaires and rating scales. These include global assessment tools such as the Health of the Nation Outcome Scales (HoNOS) (Wing et al, 1998) and specific assessment tools targeted at particular areas of interest, such as measures of medical diagnosis such as the Signs and Symptoms of Psychotic Illness (SSPI) (Liddle et al, 2002), and Beck's Depression Inventory (Beck and Steer, 1987).

The HoNOS aims to assess clinical problems and social functioning. The scales are designed to provide a rating of the worst symptoms and problems that have occurred in the last two weeks and are intended to be completed by mental health professionals following a formal interview with the client. In order to measure outcomes it is intended that the process is done at least twice to measure improvement or deterioration. James (2002) reports that HoNOS scales are used by nurses, doctors, social workers, occupational therapists and psychologists to assess and evaluate progress.

The SSPI scale is designed to assess the presence of psychotic symptoms in the areas of depression, excitation, diminished psychomotor activity, reality distortion, and insight. It is completed by professionals following interaction with the patient.

Beck's Depression Inventory is rated by the patient themselves and is a questionnaire designed to identify the presence of mild to severe depression. The patient identifies which items most accurately represent their experience over the last week and this is translated into a numerical score which is used to indicate level of depression. This can also be repeated at a later time to indicate whether there has been any change in the patients' experience.

These are just a few examples of the range of tools currently available and in use to assist in formal assessment, and practitioners need to make choices about the tools they use in order to identify the most appropriate tool to elicit the information they are trying to obtain.'

A comprehensive assessment will include an integration of formal and informal methods, producing a congruent picture of the patient's experience. It is important to use a range of assessment methods as each method obtains different, but complementary information which serves to give a deeper and more accurate picture. At the end of the initial assessment the nurse should have made a detailed description of the current problems the patient is experiencing and their current symptoms. Sources should include family and carer perspectives, and an awareness of the patient's social occupational and domestic circumstances (DH, 1999). They should also include any information from health care professionals the patient has been in contact with.

Planning and Implementing Care

During the assessment process the nurse and the patient should be working together to identify the goals for the patient's admission (DH, 1991). Priorities for the nurse may be different to the priorities for the patient.

In order to be achievable, goals need to be negotiated with the patient to encourage collaboration and engagement (Barker, 1999).

This is also the case when setting goals around the management of risk, although where there is risk to self or others protection needs to be balanced with the rights of the individual. The evidence suggests that people with mental health problems are more likely to harm themselves than they are to harm others, and the mental health nurse has a duty to protect the patient (DH, 2001). The Standing Nursing and Midwifery Advisory Committee (1999) advised that all patient's are assessed for risk of harm to self on admission. The nurse's perception of the risk to patients are more likely to include risk of suicide, self harm, absconding, and violence to others or the environment.

The patient may have differing risk priorities, including housing, employment and financial risk, stigmatisation, social exclusion, the side-effects of treatment and disempowerment in their life.

Prioritisation of goals will depend on risk levels and potential damage to self and others. Safety and the maintenance of life and physical health are top of the list of priorities.

Risk assessment and management is not an exact science, but needs to be taken seriously and be an ongoing part of the delivery of care (Doyle, 1998). The decision around the level of risk is made on clinical judgement, and should be part of a multidisciplinary approach involving all clinicians involved in delivery of care, management and treatment of the patient. Formal tools for risk assessment are available to be used by those trained to do so and, combined with clinical judgement, seem to provide greater accuracy in determining level of risk (Douglas et al, 1998).

In acute inpatient settings, the nurse's contribution has a major significance. They are a source of information for the multidisciplinary team, observing the patient over a 24-hour cycle, developing relationships with families and other carers and maintaining safe levels of supervision. Interventions designed to address risk will involve a combination of management of the environment, interpersonal strategies and medication.

A key management strategy is structured observation. This was classified by the Standing Nursing and Midwifery Advisory Committee (1999) into four levels:

- Level 1: General observation
- Level 2: Intermittent observation
- Level 3: Within eyesight
- Level 4: Within arms length.

Nurses should keep all patients under general observation and know where the patient is at all times, rising to the most intense level of observation when the patient is viewed to be a high risk to self or others.

This observation assists the nurse in their task of evaluating the effectiveness of interventions, as well as maintaining a safe environment for patients regardless of their level of risk.

All interventions need to be planned to focus on achieving identified goals and may be drawn from a range of psychological, social and physiological strategies such as medication, cognitive behavioural therapy skills, psychosocial interventions or the use of the nurses's therapeutic relationship. The nurses's role in delivering interventions will depend on the level of skill and competence, although there is an expectation that on registration the nurse will have basic skills in psychological interventions. (DH, 2006b).

Psychotherapeutic skills involve skills in relationship building, emotional management, challenging thinking and changing behaviour.

Medication management also plays a large part in the mental health nurse's role. The Department of Health has highlighted the need to enhance patient's concordance or adherence to their medication regime (DH, 1999).

The nurse has a responsibility in relation to several aspects of medication management. These are:

- Storage — ensuring medication is safely and appropriately stored
- Administering medication. The nurse should ensure that the correct medication is given to the patient, in the prescribed dose, at the right time, via the prescribed route
- The nurse needs to check that medication has been taken and keep records of this
- The nurse need to be aware of the effects and side effects of the drugs they are administering, and needs to observe for evidence of therapeutic effectiveness as well as for unwanted effects.

The literature on concordance with medication indicates that several factors increase patient's adherence to their regime. These are:

- Insight into their symptoms and the need for medication
- Involvement in the decision making process
- An awareness of potential and actual side effects
- Supervision, reminders and encouragement from others
- Perceiving benefits from taking medication
- A positive relationship with professionals, including and trusting the professionals involved with their care
  (adapted from Gray, 2004).

The above summary indicates that the nurse can be a powerful agent in supporting the patient during the process of taking medication. This may involve educating the patient around both effects and side effects, checking that the patient is taking medication and encouraging them if necessary.

The nurse's observations may confirm perceived benefits or the unwanted effects and their impact on the patient's life. The nurse may be able to act as the patient's advocate in the discussions around modification of medication, providing they are aware of the patient's point of view and wishes. The nurse's observations can act as powerful evidence to influence decisions, and assist the patient in being part of the decision making process

---

Learning Points

1. Relationship building skills involve:
   - awareness of self and others
   - reading of non-verbal cues
   - listening skills
   - responding skills

2. Emotional management involves:
   - awareness of a range of emotions and non-verbal cues for these
   - being able to name and share with patient the possible emotion the patient is feeling
   - being able to facilitate appropriate expression and containment of emotion
   - being able to facilitate the natural ebb and flow of emotion

3. Challenging thinking involves:
   - identifying limiting beliefs
   - challenging and teaching the patient to challenge limiting beliefs.

4. Changing behaviour involves:
   - identifying behavioural outcomes and goal setting
   - planning and agreeing lifestyle changes
   - teaching techniques e.g. relaxation skills.

The Integration of Skills

Nurses in acute settings are working within an environment where there is a need for a focus on both biological and psychological and social factors.

The nurse needs to develop a therapeutic relationship with the patient in order to support the patient in their experience of psychological distress, so as to gather information to help nurse the patient and ensure best quality of care from other health professionals. The therapeutic relationship offers support to the patient in taking charge of their lives and their symptoms, and engaging the patient in their own care, acting to improve their mental health.

The nurse-patient relationship is the basis for helping the patient make their own personal meaning out of their experience and helping the patient make educated choices about their treatment and their future.

In assessing and managing risk, the nurse uses the therapeutic relationship to ensure accurate and supportive strategies to maintain the patient's safety.

The acute admissions setting presents nurses with a challenge to adapt and be responsive in the use of their skills, to accommodate the individual experience of each patient in their acute mental health crisis.

References

Barker PJ (2002) Barker's Beat. *Mental Health Pracice* **5**(8): 39

Barker PJ, Walker L (2000) Nurses' perceptions of Multidisciplinary teamwork in acute psychiatric Settings. *J Psychiatric Mental Health Nurs* **7**: 539–46

Barker PJ (1999) *The Philosophy and Practice of Psychiatric Nursing.* Churchill Livinston, London

Beck A, Steer R (0000) *Manual for the revised Beck depression Inventory.* Psychological Corporation, San Antonio

Bowers L (2005) Reasons for admission and their Implication for the nature of acute inpatient Psychiatric nursing. *J Psychiatric and Mental Health Nurs* **12**: 231–6

Cleary M, Walter G, Hunt G (2005) The experience and Views of mental health nurses regarding nursing Care delivery in an integrated inpatient setting. *Int J Mental Health Nurs* **14**(2): 72–7

DH (1999) *National Service Framework For Mental Health.* HMSO, London

DH (1991) *The Care Programme Approach.* HMSO, London

DH (2001) *Safety First: Five year report of the National inquiry into suicide and homicide by people with mental illness.* HMSO, London

DH (1999) *Making a difference-Strengthening the Nursing, Midwifery and HealthVisiting contributions to health and health care.* HMSO, London

DH (2006a) *From Values to Action: Chief Nursing Officer's review of Mental Health Nursing.* HMSO, London

DH (2006b) *Best Practice Competences And Capabilities for Pre-registration Mental Health Nurses in England.* HMSO, London

Douglas K, Cox D, Webster C (1998) 'Violence risk Assessment; science and practice.' *Legal and Criminological Psychology* **4:** 184–94

Doyle M (1998) Clinical Risk Assessment for Mental Health Nurses. *Nurs Times* **94**(17): 47–9

Freshwater D (2003) *Counselling Skills for Nursing, Midwifery and Health Visitors.* Oxford University Press, Buckingham

Gray R (2004) Medication Management. In: Harrison M, Howard D, Mitchell D eds. *Acute Mental Health Nursing: From acute concerns to capable Practioner.* Sage, London

Gourney K (1996) Case Management. In: Sandford T, Gourney K eds. *Perspectives in Mental Health Nursing.* Balliere Tindall, London

Higgins R, Hirst K,Wistow G (1999) *Psychiatric Care Revisited; The care provided for Acute Psychiatric Patients.* Whurr, London

James M (2002) The use of the Health of the Nation Outcomes Scales in routine clinical practice by NHS mental health service providers in England: a summary of the findings. *The Approach* **23**: 13–16

Johnstone L (2000) What is wrong with psychiatry? *Mental Health Practice* **4**(2): 6–8

Liddle P, Ngan E, Duffield G, Kho K, WarrenA (2002) Signs and Symptoms of Psychiatry Illness Scale (SSPI) A rating scale. *Br J Psychiatry* **180:** 45–50

Mallett J, Dougherty L, (2000) *Manual of Clinical Nursing Procedures* 5th edn. Blackwell Science, London

Nelson Jones (2000) *Six Key approaches to Counselling and therapy.* Continuum, London

Reynolds W, Scott B, (2000) Do nurses and other professional helpers normally display much empathy? *J Adv Nurs* **31**(1): 216–34

Sainsbury Centre for Mental Health (1998) *Acute Problems A survey of the quality of care in acute Psychiatric wards.* SCMH, London

Sainsbury Centre for Mental Health (2005) *Briefing 28 Acute Care 2004:A national survey of acute Psychiatric wards in England.* SCMH, London

Standing Nursing and Midwifery Advisory Committee (1999) *Mental Health Nursing: Addressing Acute Concerns.* Department of Health, London

Stickley T, Freshwater D (2006) The art of listening in The therapeutic relationship. *Mental Health Practice* **9**(5): 12–18

Thomson A, Shaw M, Harrison G, Verne J, Ho D, Gunnell D (2004) patterns of Hospital Admission for Adult psychiatric illness in England: analysis of Hospital episode statistics data. *Br J Psychiatry* **185**: 334–41

Watkins P (2001) *Mental Health Nursing and the Art of Compassionate Care.* Butterworth-Heineman, Oxford

Wing J, Beevor A, Curtis R, Park S, Hadden S, Burns A (1998) 'Health of the Nation Outcome Scales' research and development. *Br J Psychiatry* **172**: 11–18

CHAPTER 7

Therapeutic Approaches in Mental Health

Godfrey Moyo

Therapeutic approaches commonly used in mental health can broadly be divided into physical and psychological approaches. According to the *National Service Framework for Mental Health* individuals experiencing mental health problems should have access to both physical and psychological effective treatments (DH, 1999).

Biomedical and psychosocial models broadly inform the therapeutic approaches adopted in mental health. From the biomedical perspective, mental illness is a result of some underlying biological pathology, thus providing a rationale for physical interventions. By contrast, the psychosocial model views psychological, social and emotional problems as an outcome of dysfunctional human responses to distressing human conditions. This chapter will discuss both of these approaches.

Psychological Interventions

Contemporary mental health professionals are now expected integrate principles of psychotherapy within their practice (Standing Nursing and Midwifery Advisory Committee [SNMAC], 1999; Barker, 1999). This increases clients' access to psychological therapies.

Psychological interventions, also know as psychotherapy, cover a number of different interventions all of which use talking and listening to bring about relief from distress. Barker (1999) defines psychotherapy as psychological treatment of problems of living, by a trained person, within the context of a professional relationship, involving removing, reducing or modifying specific emotional, cognitive or behavioural problems, and/or by promoting social adaptation, personality development and/or personal growth. Psychotherapy may be conducted with individuals, groups or families.

Psychotherapy relies on some form of interpersonal communication between helper and client, thus providing an opportunity for people to make sense of their problems and find ways of dealing with them effectively.

There are numerous different types of treatment methods used in psychotherapy, with each method reflecting theories concerning the causes of mental health problems

However, despite there being many forms of psychotherapy methods they all seem to share several commonalities. These commonalities are evident in Barkham's (2002) framework, where he identifies factors common to all psychotherapies. According to Barkham, common factors in psychotherapy can be divided into:

- Supportive factors
- Learning factors
- Action factors.

Supportive Factors

Collaboration between client and therapist is essential for psychotherapy to succeed. Individuals experiencing mental health problems are often very sensitive and feel vulnerable. Such individuals need to feel secure and protected before they can start addressing their problems. Consequently, the aim of the first encounter with the client is to start establishing a relationship which promotes trust and makes the client feel secure. This is reflected in the assertion that clients put their destiny in the hands of someone whom they hope will be understanding, protective, non-punitive and helpful (Barker, 1999). This type of relationship has been described as a therapeutic relationship and is viewed as the cornerstone of nursing practice (Reynolds, 2003).

A therapeutic relationship is a client-centred, helping relationship which develops as a result of the therapist conveying qualities which are perceived as positive by the client. The therapeutic relationship should enable clients to freely express themselves without fear of censure or rejection (Rogers, 1957). Brandon (1999) suggests that service users usually make reference to the need to be allowed to emotionally fall apart in a supportive environment. Cutcliffe et al (1997) also establish that clients value those nursing interventions that were concerned with providing emotional support.

It has also been suggested that a therapeutic relationship has the potential to influence outcomes. This therapeutic function of the relationship can be described as relationship therapy, which is a relationship in which the patient can feel accepted as a person of worth, feels free to express himself without fear of rejection or censure, and enables him to him to learn more satisfactory and productive patterns of behaviour (Kalkman, 1967).

Qualities of a Helping Relationship

There is a general consensus in the counselling and psychotherapy fields that certain qualities are inherently helpful and conducive to more successful therapeutic outcomes. Clients learn to change when the therapist is perceived as warm, genuine and empathic. These conditions are viewed as necessary and sufficient to bring about personality change (Rogers, 1957). This is further confirmed by Rowan (1983), who suggests that in client-centred therapy significant importance is placed on the therapist warmth, unconditional positive regard and genuineness.

However others suggest that these conditions merely support the application of specific techniques (Greenberger and Padesky, 1995).

Empathy Skills

This is a form of interaction in which the therapist accurately senses the feelings and personal meanings that the client is experiencing and communicates this understanding to the client. Empathy allows the therapist to get closer to understanding the client's experience rather than becoming closer to the client. As Rogers (1957) put it:

> '...empathy is the ability to sense the clients private world as if it were your own but without losing the "as if" quality.'
>
> *Rogers, 1957*

Warmth/Unconditional Positive Regard Skills

This is the process of accepting another person irrespective of their qualities or achievements. If the client feels that he/she is being evaluated the he/she is more likely to put on a false front:

> 'When the therapist prizes the client in total rather than a conditional way, forward movement is likely'
>
> *Rogers, 1983*

Genuineness/Congruence Skills

This refers to being real, open and direct in the relationship, and not 'putting on an act'. Within the relationship the therapist should be himself.

Rogers (1983) also used the term congruence to describe the match between the individual's inner feelings and outer display. He suggests that the congruent person is genuine, real integrated and transparent. Congruence allows the client to learn to trust their experience and the nurse. This allows self-acceptance, self-knowledge, self-awareness and maturity.

Questioning Skills

Question in psychotherapy is a process of eliciting information from a client about their life experience. The detail and quality of the information depends on the type of questions being asked. This can either be a closed or open-ended question.

In closed questions there is no room for elaboration. The question lands itself to simple one-word answers such as 'yes' or 'no'. During an encounter with a client there could be a need for asking such questions, for example with distressed or depressed clients. However caution is required when asking such questions as these questions could be perceived as loaded or leading.

Open-ended questions are the opposite of closed ended questions. These are questions which encourage the client to do most of the talking. They open the door for the client to 'tell their story'. More importantly, open-ended questions help to establish rapport, gather information and increase understanding. Open ended questions usually begin with 'how', 'what', 'where', 'when' and 'can you'? The aim of these questions is to:

- Raise awareness of a range of emotions and possible non-verbal cues for these
- Name and share with the client the possible emotion the client is feeling
- Facilitate appropriate expression and containment of emotion
- Facilitate the natural ebb and flow of emotion

Conveying Skills

To be therapeutic, mental health practitioners should not only possess the qualities described so far, but also be able to convey them.

Central to the establishment of a therapeutic relationship is the therapist's ability to use a wide range of communication and interpersonal skills. Talking and listening with skill is an important quality of a mental health nurse as it enables the nurse to demonstrate their understanding of the client's problem. These skills are deemed essential factors necessary for the creation and maintenance of a successful relationship. More importantly, the following skills allow the nurse to demonstrate their helping qualities:

- Listening skills: non-verbal communication of attending, remembering, rehearsing, checking for understanding and

agreement on meaning, tolerating silences, picking up on what's not being said, hunches
- Responding skills: encourages to continue, reflection, paraphrasing, empathic transactions
- Questioning skills

In psychotherapy listening is more than just keeping quiet and hearing what is being said. It involves reflective listening, which is a response to what the client is saying. The essence of reflective listening response is that it makes a guess as to what the client means. It is a way of checking rather than assuming that you know what it means. Reflective listening includes listening to the words as well as the feeling behind the words

Reflective listening has three basic levels to it, namely rephrasing, paraphrasing and reflection of feeling. In rephrasing the listener repeats or substitutes synonyms or phrases. This enables the listener to stay close to what has been said. In paraphrasing the listener makes a major restatement in which the speaker's meaning is inferred.

Reflection of feeling is the deepest form of listening, where the listener emphasises emotional aspects of communication through feeling statements. The reflection can be on the vocal tone (for example: '*I can feel anger in your voice*') or it can link feelings with the content of the message (for example: '*It sounds like you feel...*').

Used appropriately, reflective listening can serve two important functions. Firstly, the listener gains more information as reflective listening encourages the client to tell their story in more detail than they would do if they were responding to directive questions or suggestions. Secondly, the relationship between the client and the therapist develops as reflective listening promotes an open trusting relationship through empathy, acceptance and congruence.

Learning Factors

People experiencing mental health problems/mental distress may want to make some changes to their lives. Some of these changes can be achieved through learning. Collins English Dictionary defines learning as permanent change in behaviour that occurs as a direct result of experience. Learning allows the individual to grow and develop, which is what psychotherapy is all about (Rogers, 1983). Through learning, individuals experiencing mental health problems can discover more useful ways of living as well as gaining insight into the problems they are experiencing and their responses to them. Learning also enables the distressed individual to adjust to or overcome the life problems associated with distress. These changes are part of personality development and personal growth, which psychotherapy advocates. This growth and development can be achieved by nurse practitioners assisting the individual develop new insights into their life experience. Learning factors would include the following:

- Information giving
- Practical advice
- Education
- Feedback.

Action Factors

These enable the client to engage in action for change in order to remedy their difficulties. This can be achieved when the client understands the nature of the problem and goals for action.

Modelling

Modelling is a strategy based on the premises that one person's behaviour can influence the behaviour of others. This is achieved by demonstrating new ways to behave to a client rather than telling them how to behave. For example, for a non-assertive client the nurse can demonstrate being assertive and encourage the client to imitate this behaviour.

Problem Solving

Clients who get distressed or experience mental health problems because they cannot solve their problems can be assisted to develop problem-solving skills. By doing so these clients are being equipped with methods of tackling future problems. Problem solving involves seven basic steps:

- Identify problem
- Set goals
- Generate possible solutions
- Consider consequences of each solution
- Decide which solution to implement
- Implement solution
- Evaluate.

Behaviour Regulation

Behaviour regulation is aimed at changing problem behaviours and the strategies may include graded exposure and relaxation.

Graded exposure is a technique in which the client is encouraged to confront a feared situation/anxiety provoking situation in a systematic way, starting with least anxiety provoking situation working up to the most anxiety provoking situation. The sequencing of feared/anxiety provoking situation is called hierarchy, and movement up the hierarchy is determined by whether habituation has taken place. Habituation occurs when a client has remained in the situation long enough for anxiety to reduce without resorting to safety behaviours.

Relaxation could be either controlled breathing or progressive muscle relaxation. All these actions are designed to relieve symptoms of anxiety such as muscle tension or hyperventilation.

Physical Therapeutic Approaches

These are interventions which primarily work in a biochemical/biological manner. This chapter will consider drug therapy and electro-convulsive therapy as the commonly used physical therapeutic approaches in mental health.

The use of drugs is still the most common physical intervention in mental health, probably reflecting the acceptance and dominance of the medical model of mental health problems (Johnstone, 2000).

Proportionally, nurses spend more time with clients compared to other health professionals, and one of their main responsibilities is to administer prescribed drugs and medication management (Gournay and Gray, 1998). It is further suggested that nurses have a major role to play in assisting clients manage their medication and that this can be achieved by nurses utilizing their knowledge about drugs (Gray, 1999). The NMC Have produced guidelines regarding medicines administration (NMC, 2004).

The development of phenothiazines in the 1950s was hailed as a major revolution in the treatment of individuals with mental health problems. These drugs had a calming effect on the individual, hence they became known a major tranquilisers. Since then many other drugs effective in the treatment of a range of mental health problems have been developed.

Today drugs used in mental health are broadly put into groups in terms of the way they work.

Neuroleptics (antipsychotic/major tranquilisers)

These are the drugs which are used with clients with major mental health disorders such as schizophrenia and bipolar disorders. These drugs not only quieten disturbed and psychotic clients, but they also control severe agitation and reduce the frequency of symptoms such as hallucinations, delusions and thought disorders. These drugs work by blocking dopamine access to receptors. Anti psychotic drugs can be administered in various forms, orally or by intramuscular injection as either short acting or long acting. Antipsychotic long acting injection are commonly known as depot antipsychotic and their effects last between 1 and 4 weeks.

Older antipsychotic drugs, known as typical antipsychotic, include drugs such as chlorpromazine and haloperidol. Unfortunately the typical antipsychotic drugs are often associated with high incidences of side effects known as extrapyramidal symptoms. These include tremor, akathisia (restlessness), tardive dyskinesia and dystonic reactions.

Newer antipsychotic, known as atypical antipsychotics, include drugs such as clozapine, olanzapine and risperidone. These drugs have been known to produce low incidence of extrapyramidal side effects.

However, both typical and atypical antipsychotic drugs have been known to produce unpleasant side-effects such as weight gain, dizziness, sexual dysfunction and sedation, amongst other side-effects (NICE, 2002).

Anticholinergics

These drugs are usual prescribed to counteract extrapyramidal side effects, which are often produced when a client is taking antipsychotic drugs. Anticholinergics work by reducing muscle rigidity and excessive drooling.

Antidepressants

Antidepressants can be broadly grouped into tricyclic, selective serotonin reuptake inhibitors (SSRI), and monoamine oxidase inhibitors (MAOI). These drugs assist with the elevation of the client's mood and decrease the client's preoccupation with feeling of worthlessness and hopelessness.

MAO inhibitors are less commonly used due to their tendency to produce a number of severe side-effects and their interaction with other drugs and foods which contain tyramine (for example in cheese, bananas and beer). Clients prescribed MAO inhibitors should be advised to avoid certain foods.

Tricyclics and SSRIs work by blocking the reuptake of noradrenaline and serotonin, and regulate areas in the brain that manufactures these chemicals

Mood Stabilisers

These are drugs which are commonly used for the treatment and prophylaxis of bipolar affective (mood) disorders and recurrent depression. Lithium is the first choice mood stabiliser drug; however some anticonvulsants drugs such as carbamazepine and sodium valproate have been proven to be just as effective.

Lithium has a narrow therapeutic range, outside of which the drug can be either toxic or ineffective. Therefore regular estimation of lithium serum levels is required. The lithium toxicity will occur when the lithium serum level is above 1.5–2.0mmol/litre. The therapeutic serum levels range between 0.4–1.0mmol/litre (0.4–0.8mmol/litre in the elderly) (Interface Pharmacists Network Specialist Medicines (2006).

Anxiolytics

This is a collective name for drugs, such as benzodiazepines, which are used in the treatment of anxiety and anxiety-related disorders, sleep disorders and alcohol withdrawal. These drugs include diazepam, lorazepam and temazepam. Treatment using these drugs should be short-term due to their potential to cause dependence

Role of Nurse in Medicine Management

The role that the mental health nurse taken in the management and administration of medicines for the mentally ill patient is based on the nurse's knowledge of drugs. Part of his and her remit will be to monitor the effectiveness of the drug intervention.

The nurse will also take responsibility of administering the drugs safely, monitoring effects and side-effects and noting the client's response. The nurse should also adopt strategies for promoting concordance, for example, adopting the role of teacher.

Electro-Convulsive Therapy

Despite the controversy surrounding ECT, it still remains a popular form of physical intervention for mental health disorders. The negative public attitudes towards ECT have been attributed to the legacy of its early administration, where patients were given ECT while fully conscious and the confusion between shock treatments used during the war to instil fear or extract information and medical use of electricity to induce a seizure (Challiner and Griffiths, 2000). The public outcry over ECT is also linked with its abuse on political dissidents who were detained in psychiatric hospitals and given ECT as a form of punishment. The media also has not been kind in its portrayal of ECT, for example the film *One Flew Over the Cuckoo's Nest* where ECT was being used as a means of punishing controlling patients in psychiatric hospitals. According to the Department of Health (1999) 1,300 ECT treatments were carried out each week in England and Wales. This popularity of ECT is further confirmed by NICE (2003) who stated that 2,835 individuals received ECT between January and March 1999. A recent ECT survey conducted by the Department of Health (DH, 2003) established that 2,300 patient s received ECT in England between January and March 2003.

Some patients are unresponsive to medication, or find that the side effects of this treatment are too distressing to cope with. In these cases ECT may be an option.

The Royal College of Psychiatrists has asserted that ECT is a modern and valid treatment which saves many peoples lives and relieve suffering (Royal College of Psychiatrists, 2003). NICE (2003) recommend that ECT be used only to achieve rapid and short-term improvement of severe symptoms after an adequate trial of other treatment options has proven ineffective and/or when the condition is considered to be potentially life threatening in individuals with severe depression and other mental disorders.

ECT involves the passage of an electric current across the brain whilst the patient is anaesthetised. This is termed modified ECT. The electric current induces a seizure activity, which is necessary for the therapeutic effect of the treatment.

The decision to use ECT should be jointly made by the client and the psychiatrist responsible for the treatment and by so doing promoting the clients autonomy as to whether to consent or not. The administration of ECT is regulated by Sections 58 or 62 of the Mental Health Act 1983 (Section 58 is for treatment requiring consent or second opinion, Section 62 is for emergency treatment).

The issue of consent and ECT is controversial. Consent is expressed when a patient voluntarily agrees to what is proposed by the doctor and when consent can be withdrawn (Aveyard, 2002). However, when applied to ECT when a client consents and then withdraws their consent or refuses to consent a second medical opinion is sought. Treatment will then be given if the second opinion doctor certifies that the client is incapable and that the treatment is likely to alleviate or prevent a deterioration of the client's condition.

Whil ECT is prescribed and administered by a psychiatrist, the mental health nurse has a role to play in caring for an individual receiving ECT.

The Nurse's Role in ECT

The nurses role in ECT would involve supporting, educating and representing the patient, initially in the decision-making phase, and then during preparation for, administration of, and recovery from, the treatment.

Preparing the client for ECT involves the following:

- Offer reassurance by answering questions regarding the client's concerns and explain the procedure
- Ensure the client has signed the consent forms and if detained appropriate section has been completed
- Client should have nothing to eat or drink 6 hours before treatment except for necessary medication
- Remove any prostheses and jewellery, including makeup, loose teeth, dentures and crowns
- Vital signs (for example, blood pressure, pulse and temperature) should be taken and recorded
- Encourage client to empty their bladder in case they become incontinent during the treatment
- Check relevant documents (for example consent forms or detention papers)
- Apply skin cleanser to areas which the EEG stickers are attached
- Place an identity tag on the patient
- Assist the patient to get onto the treatment trolley.

Care after ECT:

- Place client on the recovery position in order to maintain a clear airway
- Monitor blood pressure, pulse, and temperature
- Observe colour and respiration
- Offer reassurance to the client
- Assist client with orientation
- Once the client has fully conscious and responding to instructions, escort to a quiet area within the ECT suite and offer drinks
- Observe the patient until client is orientated and steady on their feet
- Document all aspects of the treatment
- Observe the patient all day for side effects such as headaches and confusion.

Because of the emotive nature of ECT nurses can be left facing a personal dilemma of whether to participate or not in the administration of ECT. However, by refusing to participate in ECT nurses would be abandoning their duty to care. (Keen and Parsons 2001).

Psychosurgery

Psychosurgery is a surgical procedure performed on the brain as a treatment of mental disorders in order to increase behavioural control (Burchiel, 1983).

The procedure is rarely used now and only used as a last resort when other less radical interventions have failed (Williams, 2002). The mode of action involves destroying with precision small areas of the brain which control emotions. This is achieved by use of neurosurgical methods such as stereotactic techniques. Psychosurgery is regulated by the Mental Health Act 1983 Section 57, which states that not only a valid consent is required, but also a second medical opinion.

As with ECT, the use of psychosurgery is surrounded by controversy, mostly to do with the crude early procedures and how prefrontal lobotomy produced undesirable effects. However, current controversy surrounding psychosurgery is about issues such as the justification for the destruction of healthy brain tissues as a means of treatment for mental health disorders. Another point of controversy is that the procedures is irreversible because the neural tissue has been destroyed. Despite the safeguards of the second medical opinion provision, the question still remains as how valid the patient's consent is considering that the individual would be suffering from a serious mental health problem. Psychosurgery is a physical intervention which totally transforms an individual's behaviour, and it is therefore necessary for the nurse to offer the client support and reassurance. More importantly, the nurse needs to ensure that the client has understood the nature and potential effects of the proposed surgery for the consent to be valid.

Learning points

1. Nurses can work psychotherapeutically by applying common psychotherapy factors to their practice
2. Recently, nurses are beginning to incorporate psychotherapeutic principles to their practice
3. Nurses need to develop an effective therapeutic relationship with their clients
4. Drug therapy and electro-convulsive therapy remain the mainstay of mental health interventions
5. Mental health nurses need to have knowledge of drugs used in mental health as they play a pivotal role in helping clients manage their medication
6. Although the effective of electro-convulsive therapy has been proven, there still remains concerns over its use.

References

Aveyard H (2002) Implied consent prior to nursing care procedures. *J Adv Nurs* **39**(2): 201–7

Barker P (1989) Reflections on the philosophy of caring in mental health. *Int J Nurs Stud* **26**(2): 131–41

Barker P (1999) *Talking Cures — A guide to the Psychotherapies for health care professionals*. NT Books, London

Barkham (2002) *Common Factors in the Psychological Therapies. Principles of Psychotherapy*. The Medicine Publishing Company Ltd, London

Burchiel BN (1983) Update on Psychosurgery. *J Neurosurgical Nurs* **15**(3): 165 –8

Challiner V, Griffiths l (2000) Electro Convulsive Therapy: a review of the literature. *J Psychiatric Mental Health Nurs* **7**: 191–8

Cutcliffe JR, Dunkintis J, Carberry J, Tilley C, Turner S, Anderson-Moll D, Cooper W (1997) Users' views of their continuing care community psychiatric services. *Int J Psychiatric Nurs Research* **3**(3): 382–94

DH (1983) *Mental Health Act 1983*. HMSO, London

DH (1999) *National Service Framework for Mental Health*. The Stationary Office, London

DH (2003) *Electro Convulsive Therapy: Survey covering the period January to March 2002*. DH, London

Gray R (1999) Antipsychotics, side effects and effective management. *Mental Health Practice* **2**: 14–20

Grenberger D, Padesky C (1995) *Mind over Mood: A Cognitive Therapy Treatment Manual for Clients*. Guilford Press, London

Gournay K, Gray R (1998) The role of new drugs in the treatment of schizophrenia. *Mental Health Nursing* **18**(2): 21–4

Interface Pharmacist Network Specialist Medicines (2006) *Lithium: Mental health shared care guidelines*. Health and Care Northern Ireland, Belfast

Johnstone L (2000) *Users and Abusers of Psychiatry*. 2nd edn. Routledge, London

Kalkman M (1967) in Reynolds W, Cormack D (1990) *Psychiatric and Mental Health Nursing — Theory and Practice*. Chapman and Hall, London

Keen T, Parsons S (2000) Should nurses have the right to opt out of ECT treatment? *Nurs Times* **96**(9): 10

NICE (2000) *Guidance on the use of Newer (atypical) Antipsychotic Drugs for the Treatment of Schizophrenia*. NICE, London

NICE (2003) *Guidance on the use of Electroconvulsive Therapy*. NICE. London

Keen T, Parsons S (2000) Should nurses have the right to opt out of ECT treatment?

(Debate series. 2 opposing views on electroconvulsive therapy). *Nurs Times* **96**(9): 18

Reynolds W, Cormack D (1990) *Psychiatric and Mental Health Nursing — Theory and Practice*. Chapman and Hall, London

Reynolds W (2003) Developing therapeutic one-to-one. In: Barker, P. ed. *Psychiatric and Mental Health Nursing. The Craft of Caring*. Arnold. London

Rogers C (1957) The Necessary and Sufficient Conditions of therapeutic personality change. *J Consulting Psychol* **21**(2): 95–103

Rogers C (1983) *Freedom to Learn for the 80's*. Charles Merrill, Columbus, Ohio

Rowan J (1983) *The Reality Game: A Guide to Humanistic Counselling and Therapy;* Routledge and Kegan Press, London

Standing Nursing and Midwifery Advisory Committee (1999) *Mental Health Nursing: Addressing Acute Concerns*. The Stationary Office, London

Williams M (2002) Psychosurgery. *Br J Perioperative Nurs* **12**(12): 445–8

CHAPTER 8

Building Positive Therapeutic Relationships

Paul Rigby and James Alexander

The therapeutic relationship can be described as the central component for effective mental health nursing practice; it is the cornerstone of care and its presence is vital if care is to be effective (Rapp, 1998; Welch, 2005). The purpose of the therapeutic relationship is to effect change, and to engage the patient in any health-seeking activity the nurse must develop a relationship that is positive and purposeful.

As nurses, it has been argued that our personalities are developed and enhanced by the relationships, therapeutic or otherwise, with patients that we nurse (Altschul, 1997). Before examining the nature of therapeutic relationships in more detail, it would perhaps be useful to explore what exactly we mean when we use the term *'relationship'*.

We have all had experience of relationships, and whilst some of these are defined by our position to others as in for example, families or work colleagues, others are developed as a result of attraction or need, as in friendships. What is true of all effective relationships is that they require energy, investment, commitment and reciprocity for them to be successful and that expectations based upon role or position are insufficient on their own. For example, if we consider our own family relationships; position, as in the relationship for example between a parent and a child, does not solely define the quality of that relationship. It is the time and commitment that both parties give to the development of that relationship that ultimately leads to its 'success'.

Relationships in general are important as they help us to gauge our position in relation to others, develop and maintain our social skills, and meet a whole range of psychosocial needs (Gross, 2001). There is also evidence that the size of our social networks and the amount of social support that we receive, which will involve 'relationships' of different sorts, can strongly influence mental health outcomes positively (Repper and Perkins, 2003), and is high on the agenda in terms of what service users want from services (Repper, 2002).

Despite the acknowledged importance of the therapeutic relationship within the context of effective mental health care provision (Welch, 2005), it is a phenomenon that has received little research attention

(Repper, 2002; Hewitt and Coffey, 2005). Most research in the current climate of evidence-based practice has tended to focus upon examining the success of clinical interventions that lead directly to identifiable and measurable improvement in clinical outcomes, usually measured against a clinical symptom scale. The processes by which such interventions are delivered, such as the therapeutic relationship, is usually not the chosen area of study (Repper, 2002). However, studies that have focused directly upon the effectiveness of the therapeutic relationship in relation to improved clinical outcomes have demonstrated that positive experiences have been found to show improved treatment adherence and clinical outcomes across a range of diagnoses and treatment settings (Coffey, 1999; McGuire et al, 2001).

What Makes a Relationship 'Therapeutic?'

O'Carroll and Park (2007) distinguish therapeutic relationships from everyday relationships by the provision of a certain type of 'help' from which a person in need can benefit. Clearly, there are two perspectives to be considered here — that of the helper, and that of the person who requires help. This suggests the existence of two, sometimes competing and differing, agendas. For a relationship to be truly therapeutic, key aspects of each of the agendas need to be met. If a relationship is one-sided (thereby only addressing one participant's agenda) it cannot be identified as therapeutic.

Whilst the agenda held by nurse and patient will often differ, the perception held by each as to whether their relationship is therapeutic is crucial to its success, and an awareness of what each value in a relationship is essential.

It may be that having a good relationship with the nurse allows the patient to see the benefits of a treatment intervention such as education about their illness, help with social care issues, or even concordance with medication regimes. For patients without the significant support of a family or social structure, relationships with professionals may be a significant factor in the quality of their lives and allow them some opportunities for the maintenance and development of social kills (Deane and Crowe, 2007). For patients who have a history of experiencing 'abusive' relationships, the experience of a positive relationship with a nurse may contribute toward them developing the capacity to have safe and healthy relationships in the future (Rapp, 1998).

It is also important to acknowledge the high value the service users themselves place upon relationships that are 'helpful' (Rapp, 1998). Core competencies for mental health care workers identified by service users include respect, optimism, the ability to manage the power imbalance between service users and professionals and to demonstrate a belief in trusting relationships (DH, 2004).

In a study conducted by Rogers and Pilgrim (1994), nursing staff and in particular student nurses were highly regarded by service users, with talking, listening and the practice of relating to people in an 'ordinary' way featuring highly in their list of valued interventions.

It is worth remembering that although the context of mental health nursing has changed, in theory at least, from the more custodial settings of the 19th and early 20th centuries to community-based arenas, the relationship between nurse and patient has always been fundamental to the 'success' of care. We owe a great deal to nursing theorists such as Peplau (1988) and many others who have done much throughout the last half century to emphasize the importance of the nurse patient relationship as the vehicle for effective care (Hewitt and Coffey, 2005; Barker, 2003).

What are the Key Features of a Therapeutic Relationship?

Much of the literature refers to the principles of therapeutic relationship development, in which the key features of empathic understanding, genuineness and unconditional positive regard are promoted (Rogers, 1983; Gamble, 2006; Deane and Crowe, 2007; O'Carroll and Park, 2007).

Empathic Understanding

The ability to develop empathic understanding is an essential feature of therapeutic relationships and involves nurses developing skills which will help them to understand how it feels for the patient in their situation and to communicate this understanding to them (Gamble, 2006; O'Carroll and Park, 2007). It is not always possible to have experiences which enable us to know exactly how the other person is feeling, and in some situations it is only possible to empathize with the feelings that accompany the experience. For example, many of us will not have had the experience of 'hearing' abusive voices, but we should be able to understand the fear and distress that can accompany this experience and communicate our understanding of this to the person. This is achieved by attending to the person, listening intently, observing and asking questions to clarify our understanding. With the right relationship, both patient and nurse can work together to clarify each other's understanding of the situation and the feelings that accompany it (O'Carroll and Park, 2007).

Genuineness

The feature of genuineness within therapeutic relationships refers to the ability to demonstrate and cultivate openness and honesty within the relationship (Gamble, 2006). Demonstrating genuineness requires that the nurse be authentic, reflected in the consistency between how a person thinks, feels and how they behave (O'Carroll and Park, 2007). Crucial to the development of this aspect of the therapeutic relationship is self-awareness, with the nurse needing to be aware of their values, attitudes and assumptions and the processes at work that help to develop and maintain these.

There are professional boundaries and responsibilities to consider in this context, and whilst honesty is a necessary feature of any therapeutic relationship, professional role and a duty of care requires the awareness of professional boundaries between patient and nurse and may also necessitate the use of tact (O'Carroll and Park, 2007). For example, enquiry, gentle encouragement and prompts would be both professionally and therapeutically required when tackling the difficult issue of poor personal hygiene rather than the brutal honesty that may be employed in non-therapeutic relationships.

Unconditional Positive Regard (acceptance)

This principle dictates that all people, including patients, are entitled to care, respect and support and should be accepted and valued for who they are irrespective of their social background, previous history, beliefs, sexual orientation and ethnicity (Deane and Crowe, 2007; O'Carroll and Park, 2007). Crucial to the development of such a principle is the development of self-awareness in which our negative beliefs, attitudes and stereotypes that we hold are identified, challenged and modified for the benefit of patient care and our own personal development (Gamble and Brennan, 2006). Other key features of positive therapeutic relationships have been outlined by Rapp (1998) who identifies these as friendly, trusting, purposeful, reciprocal and empowering.

A further influential factor to consider is the context within which the relationship develops. Environments in which the client has power and autonomy can lead to relationships which are more likely to be collaborative (Rapp, 1998).

Nursing Qualities for Therapeutic Relationships

Developing effective collaborative therapeutic relationships based upon trust require patience and persistence. As relationships often need to be developed over long periods of time, insufficient time is often identified as a potential barrier as in many situations time is limited and must be used as effectively as possible (Deane and Crowe, 2007). Working with people with long-term mental health problems can often mean that an adjustment is required by the nurse in terms of not only the expectations for change but also the pace at which the change will be achieved (Perkins and Repper, 1996).

Certain qualities are consistently identified by patients as being helpful in nurses for providing the right environment for therapeutic relationships to develop (Repper, 2002; Gamble and Brennan, 2006). These include:

- Confidence, and ability to remain positive and hopeful in an environment where little or no change may be evident
- The ability to acknowledge strengths and attributes of patients
- Demonstrating the ability to address their hopes and aspirations
- Being flexible
- Developing an atmosphere of sharing and equality
- Having a good sense of humour (used appropriately).

As well as the personal qualities required, there is an expectation that the nurse will possess the appropriate knowledge base and expertise and will be sufficiently self-aware to be able to work to their strengths and utilize professional monitoring and development opportunities (Gamble and Brennan, 2006).

Barriers to the Development of Therapeutic Relationships

Although most of us are involved in forming and maintaining relationships throughout our lives, the professional therapeutic relationship provides a very specific challenge and there are particular barriers which the nurse must be aware of and overcome in order to become an effective agent of change. Some of these may involve the patient's previous, often negative, experiences of service provision which may include their relationships with professionals, the inflexibility of services and racial, sexual and cultural issues (Chadwick et al, 1996; Perkins and Repper, 1996; Sainsbury Centre for Mental Health, 1998). Furthermore, the nature and extent of some client's symptoms can also make engagement with a therapist or services and the formation of a collaborative therapeutic relationship based upon trust, problematic (Chadwick et al, 1996). For example, the natural suspiciousness that often accompanies beliefs of a paranoid nature can make the development of a therapeutic relationship more challenging.

Some of the commonly identified challenges to therapeutic relationship development are as follows:

The Establishment of 'Boundaries'

All relationships have boundaries, and most people learn at an early age that they behave differently with friends, family and strangers.

'Boundaries' define the limits of behaviour which allow a client and a practitioner to engage safely in a therapeutic caring relationship. These boundaries are based upon trust, respect and the appropriate use of power. The relationship between registered nurses, midwives and health visitors and their clients is a therapeutic caring relationship which must focus solely upon meeting the health or care needs of the client (NMC, 1999).

Boundaries are the rules of behaviour within the relationship which define the therapeutic relationship and create the space for it and keep it.

The understanding of boundaries within the therapeutic relationship is one of the most important skills of the psychiatric nurse (Schafer and Peternelj-Taylor, 2003). An awareness of the boundaries allows the helpful trusting nurse-patient relationship to develop and remain safe for both. Patients may push boundaries, trying to turn therapeutic relationship into some other form of relationship, sexual partner, friend, peer, parent figure, etc, and if the behaviour of the nurse begins to reflect any of these other types of relationships it then ceases to be safe and helpful.

There are many events in the nurse-patient relationship which will challenge the boundaries, such as lack of sufficient nurse-patient time, the patient asking for more time than was agreed, the patient asking the nurse to do something outside the allotted shift time; the giving and receiving of gifts and the use of touch. All of these can cause the inexperienced nurse some difficulty.

Meeting the Needs of the Nurse

According to the NMC:

> *'The only appropriate professional relationship between a client and a practitioner is one which focuses exclusively upon the needs of the client.'*
>
> *NMC, 1999*

There are many aspects of care wherein the nurse may be meeting his or her needs to some extent. Nurses may need to feel they are helping, being useful, that they are in control, that they are knowledgeable, and a nurse may need to feel liked by the patient. The latter is perhaps particularly evident in student nurses new to a clinical area. Student nurses also have the need to meet their objectives.

Peplau (1994) uses an example to illustrates this where she tells of a student nurse who approaches a patient on a ward; she observes that the patient looks worried and anxious. As the student nurse approaches the patient, the patient makes flattering comments about the student's hair and the student allows herself to be side-tracked into a lengthy discussion about hair care. One of the students' placement objectives is education in relation to personal care and so she feels that her discussion is 'useful' to the patient and goes some way towards her own objective achievement. Whilst reflecting upon the interaction later with her tutor, the student realises that whilst the interaction has provided a 'distraction' to the patient's anxiety and has provided her with some useful evidence towards objective achievement, she had failed to explore the reason why the patient appeared anxious in the first place.

The 'Task' Culture

There is no doubt that in-patient units are very busy places and the working day of a nurse is easily filled with tasks. Managing a ward round, running a shift, helping patients maintain their personal hygiene, writing notes, attending to physical care needs, etc. These tasks keep staff busy and give them a sense of accomplishment (Peplau, 1994).

In nursing culture there is a great deal of emphasis on 'doing something' to make the patient better, however it is appropriate to ask if 'keeping busy' is at times a way of avoiding spending time with patients, relating to them and the difficult feelings they may be dealing with. As Fabricus (1995) noted, a common coping strategy in nursing is to always 'do something' when a patient or relative is expressing distress.

The Use of 'Self-Disclosure' and 'Reassurance'

Consider the following example of nurse-patient interaction:

> *Nurse: 'How are you feeling today?'*
> *Patient: 'Not so good. I am worried about having to have more ECT'*
> *Nurse: 'You will be OK'. [Leaves the room]*

This is an example of patient-nurse communication, however, it is clearly not a therapeutic exchange as the nurse is ignoring the patients concerns and offering a fairly meaningless reassurance (*'You will be OK*).

In order to foster a therapeutic relationship the nurse must demonstrate a type of listening which goes beyond simply hearing the words the patient is saying (Stickley and Freshwater, 2006).

Below are examples of how a nurse responding to the patient's expression of anxiety could include:

1. Nurse: 'Yes, I'm a bit anxious myself today, I've got an exam tomorrow, I should be revising.'

2. Nurse: 'Yes, I know how you feel, I felt really anxious when I went in for my hernia operation.'

3. Nurse 'Yes, I think I can understand why you might be anxious, I guess everybody get anxious at times like this, I think I would be a bit worried, can you tell me a bit about how you feel when you are anxious ?'

Moyle, 2003

The first example is obviously a more nurse-centred interaction with the nurse talking about themselves and focusing upon their agenda, and whilst they are possibly trying to relate to the patient by disclosing personal information, they are not listening to the patient's needs.

In the second example the nurse is responding to the patient's needs to some extent by acknowledging their anxiety and trying to identify with the patient by once again disclosing personal information.

In the third response the nurse discloses that they also might feel anxious in the patient's situation and is trying to say that anxious feelings are normal as everybody gets them and also invites the patient to talk more about their feelings.

In all of the above examples the nurse, to a greater or lesser extent discloses, something about themselves. At some time almost all nurses will use self-disclosure, whether it is to 'break the ice' or thinking that if the nurse talks about themselves then the patient will follow suit, or that it will make the nurse seem more 'human.'

Some nursing theorists think that self-disclosure is fundamental to the therapeutic relationship, whilst others feel that the relationship becomes less professional and less helpful if the nurse shares information about themselves (Ashmore and Banks, 2003).

Not speaking about themselves at all may make the nurse appear cold, while too much self disclosure can shift the focus of the interaction to the nurse, thus adding the nurse's problems to those of the patient and also increasing the risk of emotional over-involvement in the relationship.

Another area of communication which can hinder the therapeutic relationship if not used carefully is *reassurance*. Telling a patient that things will be '*OK*' is rarely an honest response as it is something that the nurse is unlikely to know for certain, but it is an easy thing to say particularly when the patient is asking for reassurance; it can also be a way to avoid engaging the patient in communication on a more meaningful level.

It would be a more helpful intervention to explore the feelings of uncertainty and fear that a patient is experiencing. In order to use the relationship therapeutically the nurse needs to develop the capacity to contain these difficult feelings and not always go for the easy, more superficial answer.

Using '*I know how you feel*' is a common statement in everyday conversation but once again this is rarely going to be true in the case of a nurse–patient relationship as most nurses will not have had the same mental or emotional difficulties as the patient.

'*I may not know how you feel but I am trying to understand, can you tell me more*', may be more effective in furthering understanding and developing the relationship.

Communicating with patients in such a way as to enhance the therapeutic relationship often means taking the difficult option; the intervention which takes more time and requires that the nurse face the patient's difficulties.

The Concept of Expressed Emotion

Expressed emotion (EE) is a measure of the emotional climate within which a person may live, or at least be exposed to, for considerable periods of time, and which has been demonstrated to be a reliable predictor of relapse in schizophrenia and other long-term health problems (Butzlaff and Hooley, 1998; Wearden et al, 2000). The results of research indicates a clear causal link between health status and 'family' relationships, and it is now widely accepted that the quality of 'family' relationships are influential factors in relation to illness susceptibility, adaptation and recovery (Wearden et al, 2000).

Although EE as a concept has been extensively examined within the context of schizophrenia, more recently as a principle it has been applied to 'family' environments within many other illnesses including chronic depression, eating disorders, Alzheimer's disease, epilepsy and asthma (Wearden et al, 2000).

Over time, the construct of EE has been developed and consists of identified key aspects of interpersonal relationships including criticism, hostility, warmth, positive comments and emotional over-involvement (EOI), which are measured using a variety of tools, the most common of which is the Camberwell Family Interview (CFI). A high EE rating is categorised as being non-therapeutic and is identified by demonstrating either criticism, hostility and EOI alongside an absence of warmth or positive comments directed to the patient by the carer (Wearden et al, 2000).

Research has looked at EE in formal carers, and suggests that characteristics of both high and low EE can be present in relationships between staff and patients with negative effects upon patient outcomes (Tattan and Tarrier, 2000).

Health and social care professionals are being provided with programmes of psychosocial interventions to use with patients and their carers with the aim of modifying patient/carer interactions where high EE indicators are prevalent. Such programmes, combined with adherence to prescribed medication regimes, it is claimed reduce relapse rates extensively (NICE, 2002; Pharoah et al, 2003). Whilst the research to date offers slightly different figures concerning the presence of high EE levels in staff, the research is conclusive in establishing that it does exist, and can be influential in terms of patient care even if the face to face contact time is minimal (Tattan and Tarrier, 2000; Siol and Stark, 1995). Clearly, within services were openness and honesty are encouraged it may be more possible for staff and patients alike to examine the feelings behind their 'high expressed emotion' and to learn from this and adapt their behaviour therapeutically. In areas where this is less likely to happen, high levels of expressed emotion will continue to undermine the therapeutic value of relationships.

Raising awareness in professional carers of the concept of EE is of prime importance and can be achieved by a commitment to continuous professional staff development. Similarly, the inclusion of education packages focusing upon EE within pre-registration professional training is essential.

Transference and Countertransference

People respond to people based on past relationships, they transfer the emotions associated with a previous experience to the present. At times we may take a liking or a dislike to someone who we have just met if we know nothing about them, and this is likely to be based on some quality they have which we link to a previous relationship (O'Kelly, 1998). For example, a new patient may react angrily to a particular male nurse; there may be something about the nurse which reminds the patient of previous negative experiences with other male nurses, or other men or indeed a male relative.

Countertransference is a term used to describe the nurses emotional response to the patient; this can be either a response based on previous experiences of the nurse — the nurse may take a liking to a patient, but may not necessarily be aware that this is because the patient reminds him of an old friend or an emotional reaction to the patients transferred feelings.

A nurse may find themselves feeling that a particular patient is 'going nowhere and a waste of time,' and it is quite possible that this is a response to what the patient feels.

Developing Awareness of the Barriers to the Development of Therapeutic Relationships

How can nurses develop their practice effectively when faced with all the potential obstacles that can impede the development of positive therapeutic relationships? Clearly, raising awareness and improving knowledge will help nurses to recognize the potentially damaging dynamics as they develop in relationships but the provision of opportunities to discuss and explore these may also help to develop solutions.

Accessing and utilizing effective clinical supervision is essential if nurses are to dynamically develop their clinical practice in response to patient need (Dooher et al, 1998).

Much has been written concerning the factors which are perceived to influence the effectiveness of clinical supervision, nevertheless there is evidence to support the provision of regular clinically focused supervision can enhance clinical skill, develop practice, stimulate creativity and reduce stress and burnout (Berg et al, 1994; Farrington, 1995; Edwards et al, 2006).

Learning Points

1. The building and maintaining of therapeutic relationships is an essential component of mental health nursing practice and the medium through which effective care can be achieved.
2. Mental health nurses need to demonstrate skills of empathy, genuineness and acceptance alongside an awareness of the potential barriers to therapeutic relationship development.
3. The processes of personal reflection and the effective use of clinical supervision, offer the potential to examine and develop relationship building skills in response to patient need.

References

Altschul A (1997) A Personal view of psychiatric Nursing. In: Tilley S, ed. *The Mental Health Nurse: Views of Practice and Education.* Blackwell Science, London: 1-14

Ashmore R (2003) Mental Health Nursing Students' Rationales for Self Disclosure: 1. *Br J Nurs* **12**(20): 1220-1227

Barker P (2003) P*sychiatric and Mental Health Nursing: The Craft of Caring.* Hodder

Arnold, London

Berg A, Welander Hansun.U, Halberg I (1994) Nurses' creativity, tedium and burnout during one year of clinical supervision and implementation of individually planned nursing care. *J Adv Nurs* 20: 742-749

Butzlaff D, and Hooley J (1998) Expressed emotion and psychiatric relapse: a meta-analysis. *Arch General Psychiatry* 55: 547-552

Coffey M (1999) Psychosis and medication: strategies for improving adherence. *Br J Nurs* **8**(40): 225-230

Deane F, Crowe T (2007) Building and Maintaining a Recovery Focused Therapeutic Relationship. In: King R, Lloyd C, Meehan T, eds. *Handbook of Psychosocial Rehabilitation.* Blackwell, London: 57-70

DH (2004) *The Ten Essential Shared Capabilities: A Framework for the Whole of the Mental Health Workforce.* DH, London

Dooher J, Fowler J, Philips A-M, North R, Wells A (1998) Demystifying Clinical Supervision. In: Fowler J, ed. *The Handbook of Clinical Supervision: Your questions Answered.* Quay Books, London

Edwards D, Cooper L, Burnard P, Hanningan B, Adams J, Fothergill A, Coyle D (2006) Factors influencing the effectiveness of clinical supervision. *J Psychiatric Mental Health Nurs* 12: 405-414

Fabricus, J (1995) Psychoanalytic Understanding and Nursing : a Supervisory Workshop with Nurse Tutors. *Psychoanalytic Psychotherapy* **9**(1): 17-29

Farrington A (1995) Defining and setting the parameters of clinical supervision. *Br J Nurs* **4**(15): 875

Gamble C (2006) Building relationships: Lessons to be learnt. I: GambleC, Brennan G, eds. *Working with Serious Mental Illness: A Manual for Clinical Practice.* Elsevier, London: 73-83

Gross R (2001) *Psychology: The Science of Mind and Behaviour.* 4th edn. Hodder and Stoughton, London

Hewitt J, and Coffey M (2005) Therapeutic relationships with people with schizophrenia: literature review. *J Adv Nurs* **52**(5): 561-570

Moyle W (2003) Nurse-patient relationship: A dichotomy of expectations. *Int J Ment Health Nurs* **12**: 103-109

NICE (2002) S*chizophrenia: Core Interventions in the Treatment and Management of Schizophrenia in Primary and Secondary Care. Clinical Guideline 1.* NICE, London

NMC (1999) *Practitioner-Client Relationships and the Prevention of Abuse.* NMC, London

O'Carroll M, Park A (2007) *Essential Mental Health Nursing Skills.* Mosby/Elsevier, London

O'Kelly G (1998) Countertransference in the nurse-patient relationship: a review of the literature. *J Adv Nurs* **28**(2): 391-397

Perkins R, Repper J (1996) *Working Alongside People with Long-term Mental Health Problems*. Chapman and Hall, London

Peplau H (1988) *Interpersonal Relations in Nursing*. Macmillan, London

Peplau H (1994) Psychiatric mental health nursing: challenge and change. *J Psychiatric Mental Health Nursing* **1**: 3-7

Peplau H (1994) In: O'Toole A, Welt S, eds. *Selected Works: Interpersonal Theory in Nursing*. Palgrave Macmillan, London

Pharoah F, Mari J, Streiner D (2003) *Family intervention for schizophrenia* (Cochrane Review). The Cochrane Review. Issue 2, Oxford; Updated Software

Rapp C (1998) The Strengths Model: Case Management with People Suffering from Severe and Persistent Mental Illness. In: Rapp C, eds. *Engagement and Relationship: A New Partnership*. Oxford University Press, Oxford

Repper J (2002) The Helping Relationship. In: Harris N, Williams S, and Bradshaw T, eds. *Psyschosocial Interventions for People with Schizophrenia*. Palgrave/Macmillan, London

Repper J, and Perkins R (2003) *Social Inclusion and Recovery: A Model for Mental Health Practice*. Bailliere Tindall, London

Rogers C (1983) *Freedom to Learn for the 80s*. Merrill, London

Schafer P, Peternelji-Taylor C (2003) Therapeutic relationships and boundary maintenance: The perspective of forensic patients enrolled in a treatment program for violent offenders. *Issues in Mental Health Nursing* **24**(6/7): 605-626

Siol T, and Stark F-M (1995) Therapists and Parents Interacting with Schizophrenic Patients. *Int J Mental Health* **24**(3): 3-12

Stickley T, Freshwater D (2006) The art of listening in the therapeutic relationship. *Mental Health Practice* **9**(5): 12-18

Tattan T, Tarrier N (2000) The Expressed Emotion of Case Managers of the Seriously Mentally Ill: the Influence of Expressed Emotion on Clinical Outcomes. *Psychological Medicine* **30**: 195-204

The Sainsbury Centre for Mental Health (1998) *Keys to Engagement; Review of Care for People who are Hard to Engage with Services*. Sainsbury Centre for Mental Health.

Welch M (2005) Pivotal moments in the therapeutic relationship. *Int J Mental Health Nurs* 14: 161-165

Wearden A, Tarrier N, Barrowclough C (2000) A Review of Expressed Emotion Research in Health Care. *Clinical Psychology Review* **20**(5): 633-666

CHAPTER 9

The Application of Ethical Reasoning in Mental Health Nursing

John Unsworth Webb

It is perhaps because the nature of mental disorder (and therefore any subsequent mental health care) is subject to a number of different interpretations, that mental health nurses continue to evaluate and reconsider the conceptual basis on which their practice rests. Determining what constitutes good practice or a quality service, necessarily underpinned by clear ideas regarding what is being or ought to be done, can raise a number of questions both practical and conceptual. It ought to mean for example, asking ourselves what we are trying to achieve, who determines priorities and what constitutes 'good' in terms of any intervention, and such questions often create an ongoing deliberation. Fortunately, we consider this deliberation an essential part of professional endeavour where we think of our actions as being better if they are reasoned ones.

When we start reasoning about 'good' practice however, even before we get to the 'doing' phase, we are also obliged to question our understanding of mental health and/or mental disorder because how can we possibly do the right thing for individuals if we do not understand them, their situation or why they are behaving differently from us. In our efforts to understand, we recognise that the term 'health' might be usefully extended beyond the physical by its application to a mental realm, even though this means that we are already beginning to use language in a particular way which could provoke assumptions about the way things are. For example, when we talk of mental health and/or disorder we are constructing these states in a biomedical sense even though this appears to disregard the fact that neither mental states (emotions, perceptions and thought) nor the mind are usually seen in this way. This results in a position where ideas themselves regarding what might constitute metal health, and therefore our endeavour in helping individuals towards it, can appear far from consensual.

This is not so in many other areas of healthcare where professional carers and patients seem able to agree about what is wrong and more easily able to agree the type of treatment and approach which might improve things. In mental health care, such agreements are not always so easily reached, because those individuals who professional carers describe as disordered, may not necessarily agree that there is anything wrong, and where they do, they might disagree about it's cause, whether it can be considered to be a disorder, or the type of approach and treatment to be used (Dickenson and Fulford, 2000). It is where such disagreements are evident or where there is some difficulty with the concepts by which we understand individual ways of being, that reasoning, derived from ethics or moral philosophy proves useful.

The terms 'ethics' has two major elements. It is taken to mean any study of reasoning about good or harmful action, in this case related to care supposedly supportive of mental health. Such reasoning is already evident when we consider either what is meant by the terms or descriptions of mental health or mental disorder (and whether or not we feel that these appropriately describe the ways people present themselves) or whether these terms are sufficiently adequate for us to claim that a particular response is 'good'.

Ethics as Virtue

Along the way this will require us to address other elements inherent in any response and these might include aspects of our own character which we value and describe as virtues and to which another person responds. These are characteristics such as fidelity, compassion and respect for others (and because these are part of ourselves we feel that they are part of our intervention) or other aspects such as a sense of inquiry, willingness or honesty which contribute to an ethical practice. The goodness or rightness of practice also relates to such things as duty, obligation, freedom, rationality and choice, and would require us to consider any second-order or supportive terms or study such as objectivity, subjectivity, relativism or scepticism that might be associated with being ethical.

Ethics as Reasoning and Doing

'Ethics' can also mean the application of a certain way of thinking to actual practical problems, including our approach to the care of specific individuals. In the provision of care directed towards the recovery or maintenance of mental health, this might include such problems as the nature and distribution of treatment, the sphere of authority of the person using healthcare services (being careful here not to automatically label people), what constitutes a 'good' intervention, the limitations of intervention, or experimentation involving individuals.

When we are faced with a dilemma for example regarding what to do in a certain set of circumstances, what determines it as an ethical dilemma is that we are deciding on actions which are 'for the best'. This means that it is not simply a question of which shoes to wear in the morning but what might become of someone because of what we do. In an ethical dilemma we would recognise for instance that action is required, because not to act would make the situation worse. We might also recognise that opposite or opposing actions appear equal and neither obviously right. Our seeking to do what is for the best therefore means that we need some theoretical understanding by which to determine and justify our decisions.

Ethical theory is integral within a body of knowledge developed as moral philosophy and the tenets of this knowledge become evident throughout any ethical discussion. This means that we ought to be able to justify our actions or judgements in accordance with this body of knowledge even though its theories and rules are frequently tested.

Approaches to Ethics

Principalism

This approach to practical healthcare ethics described by Beauchamp and Childress (2001) seeks to apply four key principles:

Respect Relates to respect for persons, their autonomy and the promotion of self governance

Beneficence Recognises that our actions towards others ought to do good by contributing to their welfare (including their health). This includes the motivation to protect those who we see as being mentally disordered from self-neglect and self-harm

Non-maleficence This is enshrined in the phrase often used in healthcare of 'above all do no harm'

Justice Seemingly clear, this is a complex principle which arguably states that individuals should not be treated differently unless there is a relevant difference between them which justifies that treatment.

It quickly becomes evident in deliberations over a particular situation or individual set of circumstances that these principles have value related to those circumstances and may actually conflict with one another. For example, if a person were suffering from the nihilistic delusion that they were already dead and they believed that the only way to rescue themselves from this state was to kill themselves again, any attempt at suicide on their part would be rightly prevented. This means that the principle of beneficence would override the principle of respect for autonomy on two counts. The first being related to the individual's capacity for autonomy (which in this case is affected by an altered perception of reality) and the second, that death, which in this case happens to be unintended, would be the end of any possibility of autonomy as it is of everything else.

Alternatively, where a rational person sees death as the most preferable of the available alternatives, then there is a case for their autonomy to be respected (Warnock, 2006). In such circumstances, the person's autonomy may well be respected above any other concern, even that of preserving life.

Autonomy

Notwithstanding the difficulties associated with each of the principles (as well as them sometimes conflicting with each other) autonomy appears to be particularly important in mental health care. This is because whenever autonomy is neglected, the ability of the individual to develop or recover their own sense of self is undermined, and one of the key things we wish to preserve and if possible enhance in those with mental disorder, is their ability for self regard and autonomous decision making.

This is because there is a recognised connection between autonomy and substantive independence. To this end autonomous actions and choices should not normally be constrained by others.

Empowerment and Limitations to Autonomy

There are of course a number of issues surrounding the concept of autonomy that colour the way we seek to 'empower' individual users of mental health.

When we talk of empowerment, we usually mean our intent to ensure that conditions are such that an individual can act as self advocate. These conditions are brought about (and care becomes empowering) when the process of care maintains the recipient in a position where personal decision-making with sufficient support is both required and undertaken.

This position is adopted to counter the perceived imbalance of power in healthcare relationships and accepts that our conduct towards clients should respect the fact that they are in the best position to determine their own best interests as long as they have the capability.

Within this process we bear in mind that there are limitations to autonomy, for example:

- We realise that we cannot have unfettered choice because our choices might interfere with the autonomy of others
- There may be criteria to the exercise of autonomy such as rationality (being of sound mind) or having the capacity for decision making)
- We are bound by commitments we ourselves make which restrain our own autonomy (for example, if I promise to meet you at 9am tomorrow, I am no longer free to meet another individual at the same time elsewhere).

Such limitations become evident in practice in many instances especially when we try to afford autonomy/promote empowerment in those who we consider to have diminished capability to determine their own best interests.

In these cases we need to make judgements (often rapidly) regarding how best to act. Some of these are more obvious than others, for example, where an individual known to be misusing drugs, walks out on to a 1st floor balcony and climbs on to the rails around the edge; or (where we have slightly more time to consider our response) for example where an elderly client who has had an episode of depression during which his taking of medication has been closely supervised, now asks not to be treated like a child and states that he is quite capable of making decisions regarding whether or not to take medication.

In such cases, where we choose to act in the person's best interests rather than simply adhering to their own wishes or apparent intentions, we are acting paternalistically and justification for such action is grounded in the principle of beneficence.

Even though section 3.4 of the NMC Code of Professional Conduct (2004) states that 'You should presume that every patient and client is legally competent' (interpreted as meaning that the individual can understand and retain information and can use it to make an informed choice), erring on the side of caution in our decision making usually results in some degree of paternalism on our part. Beneficent paternalism supports a notion of duty (incurred within a healthcare professional role) rather than automatically promoting individual rights even though any justification for such action necessarily relates in part to the extent to which our action is judged to be therapeutic.

Individual Rights and the Duty of Care

There has been a steady move towards the recognition of individual rights for all, not least those presenting with mental disorder. Rights are simply those things which we agree to afford to one another which are sometimes encoded (Human Rights Act 2000). This means that although where they exist, they subject us to duties by which these rights are fulfilled, the claims for rights are themselves subject to judgement on the part of us as health carers and not usually simply an unsubstantiated claim. For example, if I were to claim that I had a right to see my medical records so that I could better understand how I'm being perceived by professional health carers, this would be considered to be a reasonable claim. If, however, I were to claim that I had an automatic right to certain treatments or freedoms it might be difficult to envisage how the incurred duty could be carried out without infringing the rights of others. Even so, one of the reasons why changes to mental health legislation have such a lengthy gestation is so that the power such legislation conveys does not conflict with accepted rights afforded to each individual.

Given the emphasis within the NMC's code on professional duty it may seem that care based on how we best afford rights is entirely justifiable. However, this would be a rather shallow interpretation of the NMC's intent and would make our decisions somewhat mechanistic. This is because to think in this way is to ignore the specific circumstances of each situation.

It is because situational circumstances are seen to affect the way in which we make judgements or how we justify our actions or beliefs, that there has been a re-emergence of situational ethics as the basis for deliberation.

Situational Ethics (casuistry)

In some situations, particularly where similar issues have been experienced before, the focus for deliberation can often be found using a casuistic approach (Dickenson and Fulford, 2000) which is to say, a bottom-up approach with the thinking developed from the specific circumstances of a case.

Where this is accepted, we begin to look at these related cases where there may be indicators of good or even acceptable effect from earlier decisions achievable by justified means and thereby indicative of right intention and/or right action.

It is worth noting here that there is a difference of emphasis in overarching ethical theories regarding what counts as 'good'. For 'consequentialist' theories, what is important is whether or not a 'good' outcome or consequence of an act has been achieved (Edwards, 2002). The means to this end are considered to be less important as long as the outcome is ethically or morally right. This is often cited as 'the ends justify the means'.

For deontological theorists it is the act itself which is good or otherwise (Blackburn, 1996). This is considered to be independent of the outcome to the extent that as long as our intention is good, the consequences become secondary. This might be stated as, 'the means are an end in themselves'.

Casuistry also enables us to consider whether there are elements in any related case which if altered would make our case less ethically difficult. For example, if there were a family directly involved with the rational individual who wished to die, then these might become the focal point for support on the basis that it is those who are left behind who continue to feel the effects of such a death.

This leads us into a way of bringing into ethical deliberation the issue of the perspective of others.

It seems important for example, for us to take into account the different points of view and the feelings of others who are closely involved in any case under consideration (Parker and Dickenson, 2001). After all, it is their understandings, feelings and degree of satisfaction with what's being done (elements of well-being which are themselves indicative of effective health care) which make a decision acceptable and can affect our ability to implement subsequent action. Not only that, it is difficult to conceive how any judgement or intervention could considered to be ethical or moral, and stand outside the minimal social arrangements of a respect for the way in which those affected feel (Nelson and Nelson, 1995).

Interestingly, it has been a concern based on casuistry which has questioned any automatic move away from the provision of individual client-centred care to a broader-based provision addressing say the health of a community. This is on the basis of previous experience i.e. where Nazi doctors spoke of the health of the 'volk' from which unhealthy parts (i.e. certain individuals) could be removed. (Lifton R.J. 1987).

Action therefore is not simply towards the greater good but is reflective of a general concern for the broader effect of decisions and whether or not they can be considered to be ethical. This is often stated in philosophical thinking such as that expressed by 'humanism' which although arguably not constituting a moral theory, attempts to set the necessary conditions for the acceptability of moral theories.

Humanism

Humanistic principles include a claim that the explanation and justification of the goodness or badness of anything derives ultimately from its contribution, actual or possible, to human life and its quality (Raz, 1989).

Making Decisions

When we consider whether an intervention is necessary, we are making choices about what to do for the best (including the possibility of doing nothing). These decisions require judgement about whether or how to act, and judgement must be based on some ethical understanding and reasoning.

Let us take an example of an 18-year-old girl who suffers from anorexia nervosa. Typically, although she is 1m 68cms (5ft 6inches) tall, she weighs as little as 37 kilos (5st 8lbs), still believes she is fat and avoids eating anything. When she does, she purposely makes herself sick. She has some dysmorphia (she sees herself as fat when clearly she is not) and she says things which are at best logically inconsistent such as: '*I do not want to die, but I do not want to eat anything either*'.

If we consider the type of questions this raises for us as healthcare practitioners, we can often construct the choices open to us from which we can make a reasoned decision:

- If she avoids food altogether she will undoubtedly die so should we insist that she eats? This would indicate a choice between paternalism or respecting the client's autonomy
- Her family and friends are anxious and seemingly need to be part of the treatment otherwise they might unknowingly recreate the same circumstances in which the girl's symptomatology developed. This presents a choice between individual client centredness and the incorporation of others into treatment (although these may not be mutually exclusive)
- She continually refuses dietary supplements but we might be able to get her to take them if we were to give them to her without her knowledge (e.g. put them into her drinks without telling her). This might indicate a choice between our priority for her to gain weight healthily and the treating of individuals as ends in themselves (rather than as a means to an end such as an improvement target). Here the decision shifts to one involving justice and the rights of a vulnerable person.

Reasoning Towards Action

In the situation above we might reason that it is in the girl's best interests for us to act paternalistically although we ought perhaps to also recognise the likely effects of overriding someone's autonomy (such as infantilisation or rebellion) which run counter to what we are trying to achieve.

In all health care we would wish to be doing the right thing (either to effect the best outcome or for the right motives) and this is usually focussed on the good of the individual. Mental health care however, regularly raises the additional issue about who should be the main focus of our concern – the individual, the family, the local community or the wider society (Chadwick and Levitt, 1998). This is principally because we know that the effects (and maybe the causes) of mental disorder are broader than the individual, so that even those of us who stand by have a vested interest in how such presentations are understood, how they are dealt with and what the response of the rest of us should be.

As recognised earlier however (Lifton, 1987) we might be cautious about moving too far from the principle of client-centredness in this case on the basis that care for a wider group can so easily become conflated with other things such as political desire, for example to create a greater sense of community (however laudable this might be in and of itself).

Whenever we intervene to treat individuals there is an overriding case for us to deal with them as ends in themselves rather that as a means to an end however good the end result might be generally. If we did not do so then we might begin to find justification for such things as forcible experiments on individuals for the benefit of others or oblige individuals to make sacrifices (say of their spare kidney) for the greater good.

The Ethics of Care

There is a claim amongst some nurse theorists (Allmark, 1995; Blum, 1988; Gilligan, 1982) that ethics can be expressed in a specific way through the act of care or caring which is inherent in nursing. The distinction which they make is that rather than trying to achieve impartiality through the application of abstract principles or an ethical framework, they propose that the nurse becomes involved with the other person in a subjective and sensitive manner. Moral reasoning in such circumstances, it is claimed, involves emotion as much as rationality and therefore does not look for some universal right action. Instead it bases responses on a recognition of interdependence.

It may be of course that in mental health care particularly, what we are trying to understand is entirely subjective. For example, whereas we might know certain things objectively about an individual, (for example, we can agree on the colour of their eyes and how tall they are) thoughts and feelings are not knowable in this way. It is the fact that they are only privately accessible which adds to individuality, but it suggests that an alternative way of determining whether our intervention has been a 'good' one is that instead of trying to interpret 'good' theoretically or objectively, we ought to recognise the essential interdependent and interpersonal involvement between the nurse and the service user.

Efforts to this end would then seemingly require us to work towards a shared set of values regarding what care is achieving or can achieve and this supports a circumstantial focus.

Circumstantial Focus

An example of this is that when we consider diagnostic terms such as 'schizophrenia', we find that as well as an accepted definition, they describe ways of being which are beyond symptomatology. They may for instance be partially related to such things as culture, the development of personal character and individual disposition, philosophy or beliefs. Diagnostic terms used in mental health can therefore appear to be related more to the way we as others respond to an individual and our responses in turn may be embedded in our own personal make-up, a political setting or within a point in time – for example, in the USSR prior to its dissolution, the only belief tolerated was that of communism. Because this was considered to be beyond question, anyone who believed anything different was ipso facto mentally ill, often referred to as schizophrenic and usually treated as such (Bloch et al, 1999).

Although this might seem somewhat beyond the scope of our immediate realm of care let us consider the following scenario:

Case Study

Michael, a 22-year-old, has been assessed (at the request of his mother) by mental health services and is considered to be suffering from schizophrenia.

Michael's personal history is that he came to the UK from Jamaica when he was nine years old and has had a history of unusual behaviour which became noticeable when he was 14. At this age and for no apparent reason he began regularly to walk apparently aimlessly amongst busy traffic on London's North Circular Road. He did not seem to have any regard for his own safety or for the disruption he was causing to the traffic system. This led to him receiving a caution from the police. Shortly afterwards (at the age of 15), he was found walking on one of the runways at Heathrow airport and was similarly cautioned. At this stage his home life was investigated and although he and an older sister were being brought up by one parent, their mother, (the father returned to Jamaica following divorce), it seemed to be a reasonably supportive environment. Later that year Michael absented himself from school and despite attempts to reintegrate him he never really returned.

Throughout his late teens his behaviour, manner of dress and mode of speech became increasingly bizarre and he began claiming to be in touch with God and to be receiving messages from Bob Marley (a West Indian musician now deceased). These messages seemed to order his life to the extent that he has now begun to isolate himself, rarely gets out of bed before noon and sits or lies on his bed with his body in contorted positions.

His mother supports him in his reluctance to do more and actively discourages him from going out or socialising on the grounds that people will take advantage of him. Michael himself has adopted the same stance by a benign sabotage of possible opportunities.

Since the age of 20, Michael has repeatedly taken overdoses, usually of paracetamol, requiring medical intervention on several occasions. Twice he has cut his wrists although the cuts were never deep. He eats little but smokes and drinks heavily. His sister has had some treatment for what she describes as 'stress' and does appear to suffer a degree of self-neglect. Michael's own weight is below eight stone.

His mother appears to be extremely worried about Michael but is insistent that if he is to receive treatment then it must be as an out-patient so that he can be properly supervised at home. Michael himself is reluctant to subject himself to any type of care or treatment.

Here again we are faced with a number of questions although these may assist us in the formulation of our response. For example:

- Acting differently in Michael's case may be a sign of mental disorder but it may also be a reaction to deracination and loss of cultural stability
- Tiredness may be symptomatic of schizophrenia or may relate to Michael's personal motivation (whether or not this is illustrative of akrasia)
- Self-neglect may be symptomatic of lack of motivation or an expression of individualism
- Self-harm could indicate despair and suicidal behaviour or be a personal mechanism by which to enhance reality.

Also when we come to consider family dynamics we need to take into account the potential consequences (i.e. the harms and benefits) as well as the ethics of our intent if we were to intervene to change them

Utilising the ideas expressed in caring as interdependence, we might be able to better understand and therefore more appropriately respond to the motivations or reasons for Michael's behaviour. This has importance when we consider a plan of care which necessarily takes into account our own motivation. When we express 'care intent' this doesn't ordinarily seek some uniform behaviour in Michael which might be more similar to the behaviour of the rest of us, but we are seeking to reduce any sense of distress or to promote independence where this is acknowledged by him to improve his quality of life. This may require him to more fully understand his own circumstances and by this to begin to act as an advocate for himself.

Self Advocacy

This has tended to mean not only the presentation of information towards circumstantial choice but to try to provide insights in a way in which these can be dealt with by the individual concerned and to actually increase the ability of that individual to deal with information and choice towards a better quality of life or an enhancement of life chances.

Here we begin to be drawn into a realm where we might superimpose our own values of how life might be better even if this is based on a supposedly objective view of what a good life might be.

Where we claim that a good life might be one without suffering or one in which we experience a sense of well-being (both of which seem plausible) this raises deep and difficult questions not least that of, 'Who is in the best position to judge?'.

Additionally, what if an individual makes what we would consider to be a blatantly wrong choice (or at least one with which we might disagree), for example Michael's rejection of healthcare intervention, would this automatically mean that a beneficent paternalism ought then to hold sway?

Mental health nursing implies that a particular type of nurse can provide care designed to help those with problems which we see as being related to mental health. If the title is to have meaning then we need to be clear regarding both our actions and intentions. However, as we have discussed, not only is there a difference between mental health care and helping someone whose problem both they and us understand in the same way, but we are aware that ways of being which are markedly different from those of the rest of us, can affect the rest of us perhaps as much as the individual concerned. This is in terms both of concern regarding the fate of those who can seem mentally distressed and a concern regarding what might become of us were we to succumb to such a pattern of life ourselves. Our approach therefore is one in which we seek to assist the individual to resume or comply with some state of being which they and the rest of us can find acceptable. To achieve this requires us to necessarily adopt a broad behavioural norm but also to seek to enable the other person to deal reasonably with the world and interact with it meaningfully in terms which they and us can see as appropriate.

Although such an approach may ultimately be determined as a level of preference, as the basis for our care it seems clear that continued ethical deliberation is both necessary and right.

Learning Points

1. Good ethical practice is everybody's business
2. Ethics has characteristics such as fidelity, compassion and respect for others a sense of inquiry, willingness, honesty, duty, obligation, freedom, rationality and choice.
3. Ethics can be expressed in a specific way through the act of care or caring which is inherent in nursing.

References

Allmark P (1995) Can there be an ethics of care? *J Medical Ethics* **21:** 19–24

Beauchamp TL, Childress JF (2001) *Principles of Biomedical Ethics* 5th edn. Oxford University Press, New York and Oxford

Blackburn S (1996) *Oxford Dictionary of Philosophy.* Oxford University Press, New York and Oxford

Bloch S, Chodoff P, Green SA Eds (1999) *Psychiatric Ethics.* Oxford University Press, New York and Oxford: 49–66

Blum L (1988) Gilligan and Kholberg: implications for moral theory. *Ethics* **98:** 472–91

Chadwick R, Levitt M (1998) *Ethical Issues in Community Health Care.* Arnold, London: 102–14

Council of Europe (1950) *The European Convention on Human Rights.*

Dickenson A, Fulford KWM (2000) *In two minds – A Casebook of Psychiatric Ethics.* Oxford University Press: 3–17

Edwards S (2002) Philosophy, Nursing and Knowledge. In: Daly J, Speedy S, Jackson D, Derbyshire P, eds. *Contexts of Nursing.* Blackwell, London

Gilligan C (1982) *In a Different Voice: Psychological Theory and Women's Development.* Harvard University Press, Cambridge Massachusetts

Lifton RJ (1987) *The Nazi Doctors.* Papermac, New York

Nelson HL, Nelson JL (1995) *The Patient and the Family. An ethics of medicine and families.* Routledge, New York and London

NMC (2004) *The NMC Code of Professional Conduct: Standards for Conduct, Performance and Ethics*. NMC, London

Parker M, Dickenson D (2001) *The Cambridge Medical Ethics Workbook*. Cambridge University Press, Cambridge: 160–91

Raz J (1989) Rights-Based Moralities. In: Waldron J, ed. *Theories of Human Rights*. Oxford University Press, New York

Warnock M (2006) When to die. *Observer* **07.05:** 31

See also Battin M (1994) *The Least Worse Death – Essays in bioethics on the end of life*. Oxford University Press, Oxford

CHAPTER 10

Enduring Mental Health Problems

Oduth Chooramun

This chapter presents an overview of the nature of the old institution and the effects on the clients with an enduring mental health problem. The process of de-institutionalisation and the categorisation of the long-term mentally ill clients will be discussed. This chapter will briefly focus on the transition from a hospital-based care to a more community-oriented service. There will be a minor discussion on the common mental health problems facing clients with an enduring mental illness, and the care of clients with enduring mental health problem within the framework of the recovery model embodying the main principles of social inclusion. Being positive about change and the ability of the nurse to work towards aims that are meaningful to the clients will be examined in more details. The role of the mental health nurse in the delivery of care within the framework of the recovery model and the professional responsibility of the nurse in keeping up-to-date with professional practice will be scrutinised.

The Old Institution and the Institutionalised Clients

The Mental Health Act 1983 defines mental disorders as an 'arrested or incomplete development of the mind, psychopathic disorder and any other disorder or disability of the mind', with the individual displaying significant behavioural and psychological disturbances associated with the disability. Many people are only vaguely aware of the concept of mental ill health. They have distorted images of mental illness which are coloured by fear, social stigma and prejudices. Society has often, in the past, shunned and segregated the mentally ill; many mentally ill people were treated as 'social lepers', socially unclean and were regarded as 'dangerous and unpredictably erratic' (Lyttle, 2003). The mentally ill were seen as being a danger to themselves and society, and as a result, they were kept in the big mental institution.

Mental institutions were primarily built over the past century to cater for the specific needs of people with mental illness. They were the initial creation of

'Victorian public spirit' and 'humanitarian concern' (Pilling, 1991). In the mid-nineteenth century, public concern in the 'tuberculosis-ridden private madhouse of London's east end' led to the establishment of the county asylum (Pilling, 1991). These were founded with 'great optimism' and 'high therapeutic hopes' (Jones, 1992). Community care and facilities on the scale available today were virtually non-existent. Consequently, the institution played a pivotal role in the long-term provision of medical treatment and rehabilitative nursing care to the mentally ill clients requiring long-term hospitalisation.

However, as the 19th century wore on it became more and more difficult to maintain the high level of individualised and 'humane care' which had characterised the early asylum movement. The hospitals gradually deteriorated into 'essentially custodial care (Shepherd, 1988). They became the large 'impersonal' and 'forbidding' mental institution (Martin, 1986). As demand for beds increased they quickly became overcrowded, under-funded, poorly staffed and performed a custodial function. Enoch Powell, Minister of Health in 1962, recalled visiting large mental hospitals and seeing for himself their 'horrifying overcrowding'. He recalled witnessing appalling conditions in some hospitals (Powell, 1991).

Goffman (1961) and Barton (1976) demonstrated that the environment of the institution were not 'neutral or benign' but increased the 'morbidity of the patient'. Goffman (1961) provides a more luridly expressed view on the effect of the total institution on individuals, who he describes as being 'inmates.' Goffman (1961) characterised mental hospitals as 'total institutions' where 'inmates' work, rest, play and sleep under the same roof and that the total character of these institutions is 'symbolised by the barrier to social intercourse with the outside world.' Barton (1976) points out the dreadful mental changes and effects that occurred as a result of prolonged exposure to institutional care and setting, and refers to these changes as institutional neurosis which he describes as a state of mind characterised by apathy, lack of interest, loss of initiatives, submissiveness and loss of identity and individuality. (Symptoms directly produced by a system that purported to be helping its patients.)

The introduction of psychotropic medications such as chlorpromazine and imipramine were to prove of outstanding significance to the mental health services. Clients with severe and enduring mental ill health were beginning to show signs of improvement and became manageable to the point where implementation of active rehabilitation programmes with a view to future resettlement in the community became a reality. This was further accentuated through the advent of the depot injection, which meant that less supervision were required in respect of medication administration. Moreover medical reformers also wanted to treat acutely ill clients nearer to home as they were tired of providing care in 'overcrowded' 'desolated' and run-down institutions (Murphy, 1991), supporting the development of community mental health teams. Consequently, the hospital population for the mentally ill dropped from 150,000 in 1954 to 76,000 by 1985 (House of Commons Committee Report, 1985). In addition to this, a range of community services such as day hospitals, day centres and group homes, began to develop.

In the late 1980s the climate of opinion turned very much against the large mental institution. Successive government policies for more than 25 years to run down large mental institutions was gaining momentum. As a result, in 1992 the official closure policy was launched. Closure of institutions and the resettlement of the patient in the community became effectively known as the process of de-institutionalisation. The process of de-institutionalisation was based on studies done in Scotland, Italy, Canada and other countries in the late 1940s and 1950s. The studies showed that prolonged confinement to mental institutions frequently led to deterioration of patient's mental conditions and social skills (Rosenham, 1973). Arguably, it is seen as a social ideology and its supporters hold that de-institutionalisation is desirable to the extent that mentally ill patients should live independently and that patients should assume responsibility for themselves and adapt to the rigours of life outside the mental hospital (Sands, 1984). De-institutionalisation has two components:

- Avoiding placing mentally ill people in mental hospital and the movement of those already there away from the institutional environment
- Developing and expanding community services to enable the mentally ill to remain in the community
  (Noble and Collingnan, 1987).

Bachrach (1978) reinforced this view by characterising de-institutionalisation as 'a search for functional alternatives to the mental hospital'.

In the 1980s a number of government-sponsored initiatives in Britain led to the publication of the Audit Commission Report (1986) and the Griffiths Report on community care *An Agenda for Action* (1988). The Griffiths Report proposed a radical reorganisation of services for a wide range of people with enduring disabilities to be implemented over a period of years with emphasis of shifting the traditional hospital based care to a more modern community oriented service.

Long Term Patients with Enduring Mental Ill Health

In defining the long term mentally ill patient, Bachrach (1988) put forward three criteria of chronicity to explain this phenomenon:

- Diagnosis
- Disability
- Duration.

In diagnostic terms, the long-term mentally ill client will have received a diagnosis of mental illness from an approved psychiatrist, whether as an in-patient in a psychiatric hospital or as an out-patient in the community.

In terms of disability Bachrach (1988) argues that a distinction should be made between the presence of psychiatric symptoms which are deemed to be 'impairments' and the effects of those symptoms on the individual's ability to function in everyday social roles, which is the ability to work, participate in social networking and to live a relatively independent life in the community. He refers to these as the social consequences of disability.

In terms of duration, Bachrach (1988) asserts that the mental illness has run a long course and in most cases the individual has suffered from it for more that a period of five years followed by a period of relapse and remission with guarded prognosis.

Seemingly, the definition of long-term mental illness is a product of a complex interaction between the three variables, of which the disabilities associated with the illness having a major impact.

Common Mental Health Problem in Clients an with Enduring Mental Health Problem

Schizophrenic Disorder

Schizophrenia is a severe psychotic disorder that is characterised by fragmentation of the thought process. The diagnosis is thought to account for approximately 50% of all admission to hospital, with a 1.3 % incidence rate in the population (Boyd, 2005), although the introduction of 'early intervention teams' has positively impacted upon these figures (Fahy, 2006). It is common in all cultures, races and socioeconomic groups. The gender difference for the age of onset indicates that the illness is diagnosed earlier in men that women. The onset of the illness is most common in the 15–35 year age group. Many 'outcome studies' have consistently shown that the course and prognosis of schizophrenia is poor in 50 % of the cases (Maj and Sartorius, 2002).

The characteristic features of the illness in many cases are hallucination, delusion, disorder of thought and speech, disorder of emotions and effects, cognitive disorder and a general loss of volition .

Borderline Personality Disorder

There is a high incidence of borderline personality disorder and disturbed childhood. Research findings in this area demonstrate psychological, physical and sexual abuse earlier in childhood upbringing. Clients with a borderline personality tend to have a very unpredictable behaviour. They have difficulties in terms of forming and maintaining interpersonal relationship.

This tends to have a negative impact on their social functioning, with great variation in terms of love, hates and dependency. They are generally very impulsive and do not think things out very carefully before executing them. Their mood tends to swing inappropriately. Many of them experience profound identity crisis in relation to their body image, sexual orientation, and social goals in life. Clients with borderline personality disorder have a tendency to self-harm, self-mutilate and many of them will often attempt suicide.

This diagnosis is, however, seen by many as a catch-all used by psychiatry to categorise and pathologise behaviour that is socially unacceptable.

Mood Disorders

Variation of moods in some clients with enduring mental health problems can often be severe and persistent compared with those experienced by normal individuals. The mood swing can alternate from being severely low to an abnormally high level. The disorders tend to have a detrimental effect on the clients ability to fulfil and discharge their daily responsibilities in terms of their social, psychological, physical and spiritual needs. These disorders form part of the bipolar illnesses.

Depressive Disorder

This is a lowering of mental and physical vitality to the point of distress. It is a fairly common disorder in clients with enduring mental health problem and varies from a mild form to the most severe form of depression. The clients tend to have a low mood and often may complain of decreased energy with inabilities to participate and enjoying daily activities to an optimum level and the level of concentration is generally poor. Sleep disturbance is also characteristic of depressive disorder and usually varies in accordance to the severity of the illness. The clients often have a sad appearance. In the most severe cases psychotic symptoms may be apparent with delusions of guilt, impoverishment, nihilistic persecution, hypochondriacal behaviour, auditory hallucination. Suicidal ideas are a common features in some cases.

Mania

This disorder is characterised by a period of morbid elevation and of mood, euphoria and expansive goodwill. Negative emotions such as fear, irritability, and hostility may be present in a number of cases. The clients tend to have an abnormal increase in the level of self-esteem which is often accompanied by a grandiose feeling. The clients can get very overactive, disinhibited with a high level of libido, restless, agitated and are easily distracted with a high level of thought activity present with marked flight of ideas and pressure of speech where the individual moves from one topic to another and not able to hold an idea in the mind for any length of time. Consequently, they may not wish to sleep and may think that they have a lots of very important things to attend to. The client's appearance generally is consistent with the level of mood disorder. When the mood is highly elevated, the clients tend to dress in very colourful clothes which do not always blend with the appropriate situation, and when mood is very low there is a tendency to appear neglected and untidy.

Care of the Clients with Enduring Mental Ill Health

The presence of clients with enduring mental health problems in the community have an implication for all concerned — the clients, their family carers, the various health care professional and the members of the public. For the clients, it is their fundamental rights to be able have a visible presence in the community. It is important that they integrate and interact as any other human being in the society and enjoy the same rights and privileges as others. For the carers, it is vital that they have the adequate financial and professional support. For the healthcare professionals, the availability of resources in order to deliver a care package sensitive to the needs of each individual clients within their appropriate residential settings is paramount.

The recent models of community care have focused around a case management system and assertive community outreach treatment. In the former model, the main emphasis in the assessment and delivery of care is within a multidisciplinary framework where the mental health nurse being the key worker responsible for the monitoring of the mental health of the client. The social worker has the responsibility for the social care assessment inclusive of accommodation appropriateness. While the psychiatrist will oversee and review the clients treatment as required. In the latter model, the clients will usually have complex needs and may not wish to engage the service. The main task of the community outreach team is therefore to persuade the client to comply and adhere to an agreed treatment programme.

Figure 1. An illustration of the recovery model

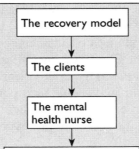

| The recovery model |
| The clients |
| The mental health nurse |

Working towards aims meaningful to clients accessing service:

1. Work closely with service users.
2. Support for other carers involved.
3. Provide accurate and up-to-date information.
4. Development of interpersonal relationship.
5. Encourage client-focused care and person-centred values.
6. Increased choices
7. Involvement of service users in assessment, care planning and care programme approach.
8. Involvement in policy review.
9. Involvement of service users in the selection and recruitment and training of nurses.
10. Advocate for the client when required.
11. Work towards reducing inequality and be sensitive to the diverse needs of clients.

Being positive about change:

1. Awareness of various changes in legislation and develop strategies to work with them.
2. Management of scarce resources in a positive manner.
3. Awareness of the wider development influencing mental health nursing.
4. Managing change and adjust to the new professional roles and relationship within a multidisciplinary and inter-agency team work.
5. A proactive approach to leadership and management in the healthcare setting that benefits service users.
6. Identify future training and continuing educational needs and update as appropriate to keep abreast of new developmental trends in mental health nursing.
7. Identify and work closely with an experienced colleague and engage in periodic clinical supervision to reflect positively on practice.

Promote social inclusion for clients and their carers:

1. Support for clients and carers.
2. Facilitate development of social links.
3. Valued social roles for clients in society.
4. Encourage prospects of employment, education, and training opportunities.
5. Works towards reducing social stigma attached to mental illness.
6. Promote concept of mental health and health promotion with youngsters in school and colleges.
7. Use of unused school facilities to enhance discussion, seminars and meetings and set up small activities in groups involving clients.

All team members have the same level of input in the delivery of care and the overall responsibility is shared by the whole team.

However, the recovery model (see *Figure 1*) is an interesting conceptual framework for delivering future care and intervention package to clients with enduring mental illness. The Chief Nursing Officer's review of mental health nursing *From Values to Action* (DH, 2006) clearly endorsed this view. It is stated that mental health nursing 'should incorporate the broad principles of the recovery approach into every aspect of their practice' (DH, 2006). The report states that the mental health care professionals should move more in the following direction:

- Towards aims that are meaningful to the clients accessing the service
- Being positive about change
- To promote social inclusion for the clients and their carers.

The Role of the Mental Health Nurse: Embodying the Broad Principles of the Recovery Model

Aims that are Meaningful to Service Users

It is important that clients suffering with enduring mental health problems are adequately supervised, monitored and assisted to access services and treatment facilities. These facilities should be locally available and the clients should be provided with sufficient information to make informed decisions about their care; for example reaching concordance with regard to decisions about medications.

The delivery of care has to be sensitive to the needs of the diverse group of clients in our modern society. Service users need to feel valued as members of the society who have an important role to play not only in relation to their own care delivery but encouraged to fulfil a valued social role so that a positive perception of them emerges. Meaningful involvement of the client, their family, carers and partners in the making of decisions which impact upon care is an important step in achieving this aim.

Clients with enduring mental health problems have a right to seek and access services that are available. The range of services that are available should therefore be 'accessible' to the mentally ill clients and 'appropriate to the needs of the whole community.' Gelder et al (2005) state that services for the mentally ill should be effective, efficient, economical, equitable and acceptable to the clients. The facilities should be made available to the clients irrespective of their disability, colour, creed, religion and their diverse cultural orientation. This is consistent with the influence of the Human Right Act 1998 which clearly establishes the prohibition of discrimination . It is thus imperative that people with disability should enjoy the same privileges and rights when come to have accessing the range of services in society. Hence respecting the clients wishes, aspiration, their specific need for services at the point of delivery is important. The clients ability in making decision in relation to their own care planning; encouraging them in mobilising resources to solve their own problems and meeting their own needs and recognising their human rights is an important aspect of empowerment that need to be transparent in the process of care delivery. A partnership has to be formed between the client and the nurse that takes into consideration of the various aspects cited above. Thus the active involvement of the clients in their design and implementation of the agreed care plan is paramount.

It is also very important that the mental health nurse enhances the concept of a holistic approach to the care of the client. This mean that the client is seen as a whole individual who, irrespective of their psychological and mental health problem, still have other diverse needs in the realms of physical, social and spiritual dimension that will require a robust assessment and a creative intervention from the nurse practitioner. A holistic approach that stresses the value of a holistic perspective is crucial in trying to understand the individual as a whole, his/her health in general and his/her subsequent illness. Consideration should also be given to the political and economic factors influencing the client's wellbeing.

The delivery of culturally appropriate services that take account of the cultural context of the client background should also form part of the holistic care approach. The skill of the mental health nurse in making a holistic assessment of the clients' needs is therefore a key factor in compiling a realistic assessment of the diverse needs of the clients. There may be risk factors that need to be identified and subsequently managed appropriately. Identifying any potential risk is an important aspect of care and management with clients of enduring mental health problem who are suitable for community living. Risk assessment is a critical element in the planning and delivery of quality care. It is an aspect of good clinical practice. McInnes (2000) argues that an important role of the mental health nurse is to assess the risk that people with mental illness pose to themselves and to others. Risk assessment is viewed as a critical skills in the *National Service Framework for Mental Health* (DH, 1999). Risk assessment and management should be carried out within the framework of a multidisciplinary team approach.

The value of delivering care to clients with enduring mental health problem within the framework of a multidisciplinary team has benefits for all concerned. Payne (2000) states that 'multidisciplinary and inter-agency work imply respectively that several potential groups with various knowledge and skill base are drawn together in a structure to provide services. This is supported by the Department of Health (DH, 2000), which advocates multidisciplinary and inter-professional working as the way forward for modern health and social care. Good mental health practice is all about working effectively and in partnership with others, and is a good example of providing seamless quality care for the clients.

The nurse has to be proficient in using reliable tools and demonstrate the required specific skills in order to be able to produce more realistic assessment information and data on the clients psycho-bio-social state. The involvement of the clients themselves and their representatives in the very design of the care planning and delivery is an important part of the equation. This will lead to an increase level of service user involvement, choices and decision-making.

Being Positive about Change

The environment faced by the NHS is rapidly changing. The emphasis on cost and the demand on delivery of a quality care package is becoming more and more robust in all areas of health care. Nurses are operating in a more proactive and competitive circumstances where they have to be aware of changes in service users needs and preferences and the availability of resources in their own department. Mental health care professionals have to be capable of reacting to their rapidly changing environment and focus more clearly on how to manage the change effectively. The nurses have to be able to manage the current changes occurring in the health service and the society in general with some degree of challenge, creativity and innovation if they are to be in a position to deliver comprehensive care package to clients in the new modern arena with rapid social and technological changes.

The current political climate in the country must be taken into consideration in the planning and implementation of care and services for the clients with an enduring mental health problem. It is clear that resources will not be available in excess of what is strictly required. Therefore, making use of scarce resources available in order to satisfy wants and needs is an important philosophical consideration that the nurse should bear in mind. Being able to manage the scarce resources in order to achieve the primary objectives for management and the clients is the future challenge and changes facing the nurse.

Promoting Social Inclusion

Education and the promotion of mental health and the integration of the clients in the community and the public awareness of this is crucial in sustaining the clients in the community after discharge. The concept of stigma, social exclusion and discrimination have impact on the delivery of services. For the public, it is important that they see the community integration of the clients and their continued presence in the community as a normal development in the delivery of care to clients with enduring mental ill health. The need to reduce the level of social stigmatisation, discrimination and enhancing the concept of social inclusion is an important step forward in the long term care of the clients. It is argued the changes in the way mentally ill people are perceived and the enhancement of a valued social role for the clients in line with the philosophy of social role valorisation will greatly assist in the integration of a meaningful coexistence in the community (Wolfensberger, 1993).

More recently this aspiration has been supported by the government by a range of publications from the Social Exclusion Unit (DH, 2004), and the development of the National Social Inclusion Programme. These have bought together organisations in a 'concerted effort' to challenge attitudes, enable people to fulfill their aspirations, and significantly improve opportunities and outcomes for people with mental health problems. The report sets out a 27-point action plan which fall into six categories:

- **Stigma and discrimination**: a sustained programme to challenge negative attitudes and promote awareness of people's rights
- **The role of health and social care in tackling social exclusion**: implementing evidence-based practice in vocational services and enabling re-integration into the community
- **Employment**: giving people with mental health problems a real chance of sustained paid work reflecting their skills and experience
- **Taking part in local community**: enabling people to lead fulfilling lives the way they choose
- **Getting the basics right**: access to decent homes, financial advice and transport
- **Making it happen**: clear arrangements for leading and maintaining programme momentum

The therapeutic use of work and leisure activities in the promotion of mental health for the clients will accentuate the process of independent community living. Hence encouraging clients to make effective use of various recreational and leisure facilities within the community will encourage active integration within the community. This is a crucial point of consideration in the provision of care to clients with enduring mental health problem. Both the clients and their respective carers should be encouraged to access the range of services available irrespective of their disability, gender, race, creed, culture and religion. The Disability Discrimination Act of 1995 makes it specifically clear that the underprivileged and disabled people have the right to access the range of services available to them and that the service provider has to make the service easily accessible. It is therefore important that service providers should take into careful consideration the client's whole situation in terms of their social entourage, family, significant others, housing, education, employment, social, cultural diversity, work and leisure pursuit, religious and spiritual needs. Removing discriminatory barriers and enabling the clients with mental health disability to feel valued will inevitably facilitate the development of a valued social role for the clients in the community care arena. This has the potential to accentuate the process of integration and will help to question the social role perception of the mentally ill in the community.

The nurse working within a holistic framework will be able to focus more clearly on the social process of devaluation and take this into consideration in the assessment and planning process so that the needs of the enduring mentally ill clients are realistically met. Moreover, proper assessment of families and carers needs so that a cluster of flexible support services could be developed and made available is a positive step forward. Inevitably, the nurse will have to see it as their ultimate responsibility to ensure that the quality of information the clients, their families and carers receive on the range of services presented is accurate and reliable. Accurate and readily available information on available services is the key equation in the provision of care to clients with enduring mental health problem in modern days. Technological advances together with the advent of home computers and the easy access and spread of e-mails and Internet services means that service users are now able to access a range of information on services currently on offer to meet their diverse needs. One of the main aims of good practice within the framework of a holistic care approach is to increase the service users awareness of the various range of treatment and therapeutic modalities currently available to them and how best they can access them whenever required.

The question of social stigma attached to mental illness has to be addressed effectively. Programmes on community education and mental health promotion activities aimed at youngsters in school and colleges and community health centre about mental illness and how it affects the individual has to be undertaken on a regular basis. This should be done in partnership with other disciplines and the service users in order to increase public awareness of the difficulties, hostilities and labelling that mentally ill clients encounter from time to time in the community. Effecting attitude change in people in relation to a more positive and tolerant behaviours towards the plight of the mentally ill in the community would produce a significant impact on breaking down the social stigma and barriers attached to mentally ill. The inclusion of people with mental health problem, their respective representatives and their advocacy in the consultation initiatives by statutory bodies and encouraging decision making on planning and implementation of care package sensitive to their needs are a good example of positive practice. It is also a good means of promoting user involvement and widening participation and decision making in the very design and delivery of care.

Professional Development for the Nurse

The NMC *Code of Professional Conduct* (NMC, 2004) clearly states that qualified nurse practitioners are personally accountable for their practice. Therefore in the process of caring for their clients, they have a moral responsibility to maintain their professional knowledge and competence. To do this effectively and professionally well, nurses have a duty to equip themselves with the appropriate skills and knowledge at the time of delivery. It is thus important for the nurse practitioners to keep their 'knowledge and skills up-to-date throughout their working life' (NMC, 2004). The maintenance of a professional development portfolio that addresses current competence, deficit in skills, knowledge and the seeking of the appropriate training in order to keep abreast of developmental trend in their specialist area is a crucial activity that should be undertaken jointly within the framework of sound clinical supervision.

Learning Points

1. There are three criteria of chronicity to define the long-term mentally ill patient: diagnosis, disability and duration.
2. The presence of clients with enduring mental health problems in the community have an implication for all concerned — the clients, their family carers, the various health care professional and the members of the public.
3. The concept of community supervision, and adequate contact with the clients in order that they are able to access the services and treatment facilities available, together with medication concordance, are crucial factors that need to be taken into consideration in order that the process of continued recovery and the prevention of relapse in the community is sustained.
4. Clients with enduring mental health problems have a right to seek and access services that are available.

References

Audit Commission Report (1986) *Making a reality of community care*. HMSO, London

Bachrach L (1978) A conceptual approach to de-instituitionalisation. *Hospital and community psychiatry* **29:** 573

Bachrach L (1988) Defining chronic mental illness: A concept paper. *Hospital and community psychiatry* **39:** 383–8

Barton R (1976) *Institutional Neurosis*. Wright, Bristol

Boyd MA (2005) *Psychiatric nursing – Contemporary practice*. Lippincott Williams & Wilkins, Publication

DH (2006) *From Values to Action: Chief Nursing Officer's review of mental health nursing*. DoH,

DH (2000) *Journey to Recovery. The Government Vision for Mental Health Care*. HMSO, London

Fahy M (2006) Early intervention in psychosis. In: Dooher J, ed. *New Ways of Working in Mental Health*. Quay Books, London

Gelder M, Mayou R, Geddes J (2005) *Psychiatry*. 3rd edn. Oxford University Press, Oxford

Goffmann I (1961) *Asylums*. Penguin Publication, London

Griffiths R (1988) *Community Care: An Agenda for Action*. HMSO, London

House of Common Committee Report (1985) *Second Report from Social Services Committee: Community care with special reference to mentally ill and mental handicapped people*. Stationery Office, London

Jones K (1992) *A History of the Mental Health Services*. Routledge and Kegan Publications, HMSO, London

Lyttle J (2003) *Mental Disorders: Its Care and Treatment*. Balliere Tindall, London

Maj M, Sartorius N (2002) *Schizophrenia. WPA series: Evidence and Experience in psychiatry*. Jon Wiley & sons Ltd, Sussex

Martin J (1986) *Hospital in Trouble*. Blackwell Publication, Oxford

McInnes D (2000) *Assessmant of Risk Posed by People with Mental Illness*. NT Monographs. NT Emap Health Care Ltd, London

Mental Health Act (1983) Her majesty's Stationery office, London

Murphy E (1991) *After the Aylums – Community care for people with mental illness*. Faber & Faber publication Ltd, London

NMC (2004) *The NMC code of professional conduct: standards for conduct, performance and ethics*. NMC, London

Noble J, Collignan F (1987) Systems barriers to support employment for persons with chronic mental illness. *Psychosoial R Rehabilitation Journal* **xi**(2): 56

Payne S (2000) *Teamwork in Multi-Professional Care*. Macmillan Publication, Basingstoke

Pilling S (1991) *Rehabilitation and Community Care*. Routledge Publications, London

Powel E (1991) In: *After the Asdylums – Community care for people with mental illness*. Murphy E, ed. Faber and Faber, London

Rosenthan D (1973) On being sane in insane places. *Science* **179:** 250–8

Sands D (1984) ' Correlates of success and lack of success in community de-institutionalisation. *Community Mental health Journal* **120:** 223–35

Shepherd G (1988) *Current Issues in Community Care*. Paper given at Annual conference on Rehabilitation of psychiatric patients and their care in the community. Randolph Hotel, Oxford, 13.12.88

Social Exclusion Unit (2004) *Mental Health and Social Exclusion*. DH, London

Wolfensberger W (1993) *Social Role Valorisation: Proposed new term for the principles of normalisation*. Routledge, London

CHAPTER 11

The Relationship Between Physical Health and Mental Health

Jacqui Day

Anyone who takes even a cursory interest in health news will be aware of an increasing emphasis on the physical health needs of the nation. However, while the risks of obesity, diabetes and heart disease for the population in general seem to be increasing at an unacceptable rate, the risks for some groups, in particular those members of the population who suffer some form of mental illness and/or distress, are even greater.

Under the weight of evidence, originally conducted 10 years ago, the view that individuals with mental health problems have higher rates of physical illness, resulting in a higher death rate, still retains currently, and while psychiatry continues to have a stronger association with unnatural death than other branches of medicine, death from natural causes is at least as significant (Harris and Barraclough, 1998). It is estimated that natural deaths account for 59% of the excess mortality compared to 28% for suicide in patients with schizophrenia (Le Fevre, 2001).

There are many possible factors contributing to this, including lifestyle, socio-economic position, the stigma leading to social exclusion and the often detrimental, iatrogenic, effects of diagnosis and subsequent treatments (NIMHE, 2004a). This chapter will explore the evidence leading to these conclusions and look at some of the opportunities available to redress the balance.

Physical Health Risks

The increased physical health risks for people who experience mental distress relate to a range of conditions including endocrinal, gastrointestinal, respiratory and coronary heart disease, diabetes and infections, of course, can have a detrimental effect on mental health (Mentality and NIMHE, 2004c). Individuals with a mental disorder are twice as likely to die from coronary heart disease as the general population, and more specifically adults with severe or enduring mental health problems such as those with a diagnosis of schizophrenia, psychosis or bi-polar disorder are four times more likely than those without a mental illness to die from respiratory infections and/or disease (Phelan et al, 2001; Cohen and Hove, 2001; Mentality and NIMHE, 2004c).

An adult with schizophrenia can expect to live ten years less than non-schizophrenic counterparts, and is significantly more likely to experience a greater incidence of circulatory disorders, digestive diseases, diabetes and bowel cancer (Baxter, 1996; Brown et al, 2000; Disability Rights Commission, 2006).

Women with schizophrenia are 42% more likely to develop breast cancer than other women (Disability Rights Commission, 2006). As if this was not enough, service users who experience significant weight gain can also add an increased risk of type 2 diabetes, hypertension, cardiovascular disease, osteoarthritis and some types of cancer to their list (Goldman, 1999).

Of course, one of the most frustrating aspects of this is that most of these conditions are largely preventable and/or responsive to treatment and other interventions. However, many of these conditions frequently go undetected (Phelan et al, 2001). Ironically, the GP consultation rate for individuals who use mental health services is significantly higher than average, standing at 13-14 consultations per year compared with an average consultation rate of 3-4 (Mentality and NIMHE, 2004c).

Kendrick (1995) studied 101 people living in the community with a severe and enduring mental health problem and found that although conditions such as hypertension, shortness of breath, wheezing, chest pain and coughs producing sputum were significantly more common in the study group than in a comparative population group, there were few attempts to intervene. There is further evidence to support the view that generally the physical health needs of individuals with mental health difficulties are largely ignored by professionals (Mentality and NIMHE, 2004c; Roberts et al, 2007). It has also been suggested that mental health service users are less likely to be offered health promotion advice with regards to smoking, alcohol, diet and exercise and receive blood pressure, cholesterol, urine or weight checks (Mentality and NIMHE, 2004c). (However there is some evidence to suggest that this is problem is now being addressed through the new General Medical Council contracts (Disability Rights Commission, 2006).)

Reasons for Poor Physical Health in People with a Mental Illness

It is likely this situation results from a range of factors. Phelan et al (2001) suggest it might be the impact of avoidance from some health professionals who are inexperienced, or uncomfortable, with mental health issues. Fear, prejudice and inadequate communication skills can compromise a successful health relationship, particularly with individuals whose presentation results in behavioural disturbances such as hostility, communication deficits, violence and aggression (Standing Nursing and Midwifery Advisory Committee, 2005).

There is also the possibility that experienced mental healthcare professionals lack relevant experience, and knowledge, of physical health issues and/or attribute physical symptoms to a psychological cause (diagnostic overshadowing).

Service users frequently complain that once a psychiatric diagnosis is made, any physical health concerns are considered to be further evidence of psychiatric illness (Dean et al, 2001; Mentality and NIMHE, 2004c; Forrest, 2006).

The situation is further compounded by the fact that although a third of service users listed regular physical health checks as one of their top three priorities (Rethink, 2003) research indicates that individuals with schizophrenia are less likely than healthy controls to report physical symptoms spontaneously (Jeste et al, 2001). This could be due to several factors, for example, the impact of the residual symptoms of schizophrenia such as poor motivation, a change in cognitive functioning and social withdrawal, disempowerment and lack of confidence as a consequence of stigma and increased levels of social exclusion and marginalisation, and finally the reactive, rather than preventative, nature of the health care system in general (Phelan et al, 2001).

However, this in itself is not enough to explain the physical health inequalities experienced within this group and other contributory factors need also to be taken into account.

Individuals who experience mental health disorders generally tend to have unhealthier lifestyles than other comparative population groups. They tend to smoke more, eat poorer diets, and take less exercise (Mentality and NIMHE, 2004c; Robson and Gray, 2005). Incidences of substance abuse, including alcohol, cannabis, psychoactive and intravenous drugs are also significantly raised, particularly in individuals who experience a severe and enduring mental health illness such as schizophrenia (Goldman, 1999).

Diet

Poor diet is implicated in a range of conditions including cardiovascular disease, certain cancers, obesity and type 2 diabetes.

It has been suggested that many individuals with a severe and enduring mental illness frequently have an insufficient and unbalanced diet compared with the rest of the population. This results in significantly lowered intake of fibre and essential, protective antioxidant vitamins in addition to raised intakes of saturated fat (Brown et al, 1999). Consumption of fruit and vegetables are often well under the recommended daily intake, but according to the Mental Health Foundation's (2006) recent national opinion poll less than half of respondents who reported daily mental health problems eat fresh fruit, vegetables or juice on a daily basis, compared with two thirds of respondents who do not experience mental health problems. Of course, this is not just limited to people living in the community, poor nutrition is also a recognised problem for the in-patient population who often find themselves at the mercy of inflexible and interrupted mealtime arrangements, unappetising or inappropriate food, poor quality catering, and inadequately educated nursing and medical staff (Dickinson et al, 2004).

Not surprisingly, this corresponds with increased levels of obesity. It is reported that 33% of people with schizophrenia and 30% of people with bi-polar disorder are obese, compared with 21% of the general population (Disability Rights Commission, 2006).

Smoking

Rates of smoking are also significantly raised in people with mental health illness. It is estimated that 61% of people with schizophrenia and 46% of those with bi-polar disorder smoke, compared with 33% of the general population (Disability Rights Commission, 2006). People with mental health illness are also more likely to be classified as heavy smokers, smoking 25 or more cigarettes a day (McCreadie, 2002). Smoking is particularly prevalent in (psychiatric) in-patient facilities (Rethink, 2003), especially in patients with a psychotic disorder (Mentality and NIMHE, 2004c). However it is suggested that this could be as a result of boredom and a lack of alternative pastimes (Dean et al, 2001).

Although there is no dispute about the detrimental relationship between smoking and physical health, the relationship between smoking and mental health is more complex. Smoking behaviour has a lengthy association with the culture of psychiatric institutions (Robson and Grey 2005), which may offer some explanation as to why smoking cessation programmes are often noticeably absent in these environments (Disability Rights Commission, 2006), although this may change in response to recent smoking legislation (DH, 2007).

There is some speculative evidence to suggest that smoking might alleviate negative symptoms such as social withdrawal and flattened affect, reduce the side effects of antipsychotic medication, such as parkinsonism and sedation, and improve cognitive functioning and concentration in people with schizophrenia. As is the case in the use of other addictive substances there are also complex social aspect to the behaviour. Some studies suggest that people with schizophrenia smoke to relax, for pleasure and/or as a way of making social contact. When a smoking habit is part of a daily routine it can also provide essential structure and purpose to the day (Robson and Gray, 2005).

However, despite some of the apparent benefits, there is contradictory evidence that indicates that because of the increased dopaminergic activity that nicotine causes, smoking can have a negative impact on mental health, contributing, for example, to the development of anxiety states, depression and perhaps other mental disorders (Rethink, 2003). In addition, the hydrocarbon agents in tobacco have been found to increase the metabolism of antipsychotics which, by necessitating higher doses to achieve the desired effect, actually increases the chances of side effects (Robson and Gray 2005).

Alcohol and Substance Misuse

Adults with a diagnosis of schizophrenia are more likely to misuse substances than the remainder of the population. It has been suggested that between 20–70% of people with schizophrenia use a variety of substances — ranging from marijuana, intravenous drugs and alcohol — at some point in their lives and are more frequent users of psychoactive drugs and stimulants (Mentality and NIMHE, 2004c).

Although alcohol and substance misuse has often used as a way of managing, or minimising, symptoms, the negative impact on mental health is also apparent, for example, a recent study which links the use of cannabis with an increased risk of developing psychosis (Mentality aand NIMHE 2004c).

Exercise

Sedentary habits account for a significant proportion of deaths due to coronary heart disease, type 2 diabetes and colon cancer, and has been identified as an independent risk factor for cardiovascular disease.

Individuals with mental health difficulties are more likely to have sedentary lifestyles than the general population, possibly due to lack of motivation and/or opportunity (Mentality and NIHME, 2004c; Faulkner and Taylor, 2005).

Inactivity, along with boredom, is also a factor identified in studies of hospital life (Dean et al, 2001).

Stress

There is an increasing body of evidence which demonstrates the negative impact of stress on physical processes such as cholesterol metabolism, blood pressure, blood clotting and platelet aggregability, diabetes and immunity against infectious and autoimmune diseases and cancer (Mentality and NIMHE, 2004c). Chronic or long-term stress is also thought to cause neuronal deterioration and peptic ulceration, not to mention the exacerbation of mental disorders such as anxiety and depression. Of particular concern is the evidence which demonstrates that children who experience extreme, and/or persistent stress, for example as a response to abuse or severe emotional deprivation, can experience direct and permanent damage to the developing brain which can result in depression, withdrawal, suicidal tendencies, anxiety, anger, aggression, delinquency, unstable relationships and personality disorders in later life (Blows, 2003).

Although the primary biological pathway linking stress with physical disease is thought to be hormonal, behavioural responses to stress also need to be considered. For example, individuals who are under stress may drink more alcohol, smoke more, experience an alteration in appetite, take less exercise and suffer disturbed sleep patterns (Cohen et al, 1995).

Individuals who experience mental disorders are often more vulnerable to stress due to experiences of stigma and social exclusion contributing to isolation, insecurity, low self esteem and paternalistic attitudes from professionals resulting in a lack of personal control and responsibility (Dean et al, 2001; Mentality and NIHME, 2004a).

Medication

Weight gain is a known side-effect of most psychotropic medications, including for typical and atypical anti-psychotics, antidepressants and mood stabilisers (Stahl, 2000; Pulzer, 2006). While this problem is not limited exclusively to this population group, compared with the general population, individuals with severe and enduring mental health diagnoses are more likely to be overweight, or obese. This risk is further increased in the 30% of individuals who do not respond to standard anti-psychotics and who often receive both higher doses and a combination of drugs (National Schizophrenia Fellowship, 2001). Not only does weight gain lead to an increased risk of physical disorders such as type 2 diabetes and heart disease, but the psychological effects can also be profound; next to sedation and lethargy, weight gain has been ranked as one of the most troubling side-effects by service users leading to a reduction in self esteem and self confidence (Dean et al, 2001).

Hyperglycaemia has long been associated with traditional phenothiazine derivatives, loxapine and the antidepressant amoxapine (Mir and Taylor, 2001). There is now an increasing body of evidence to suggest that atypical, or second generation, anti-psychotics, in particular clozapine and olanzapine, can also be linked with impaired glucose tolerance resulting in hyperglycaemia, diabetes mellitus and/or diabetic ketoacidosis, abdominal weight gain (central obesity), reduced HDL cholesterol, raised triglyceride and elevated blood pressure. Collectively referred to as metabolic syndrome, these symptoms are also associated with an increase in cardiovascular disease (Pulzer, 2006; Usher et al, 2006; Law, 2007).

A further detrimental effect of anti-psychotic medication, with the exception of clozapine and quetiapine in this case, is the potential for pathologically elevated prolactin levels resulting in reduced bone mineral density and an increased risk of osteoporosis (Meaney et al, 2004). Another possible side-effect of various anti-psychotics, although significantly less common amongst the atypicals, includes a potential for cardiotoxity which can result in sudden death (National Schizophrenia Fellowship, 2001; Marder et al 2004).

Extra-pyramidal symptoms, such as inner restlessness, muscle spasms, tremors and shaking, are a particularly troubling side effect commonly associated with typical anti-psychotic medication effecting up to 75% of people who take them. These unwanted effects can cause extreme distress, worsen psychotic symptoms and increase suicide risk and non-concordance. Over-sedation and lethargy and sexual dysfunction are also included in service users experience of anti-psychotic medication, which again can have a profound effect on quality of life, self perception and the ability to engage with social and emotional aspects of living (National Schizophrenia Fellowship, 2001).

Although medication has undoubted benefits, the unwanted effects of many psychotropic medications can further complicate the already compromised physical health outcomes of people with mental illness, particularly those with a more severe and enduring presentation.

Socio-Economic Position

The link between a disadvantaged socio-economic position and poor health outcomes, both physical and mental, is well established (Graham, 2004). This is mediated and influenced through environmental and psychosocial factors such as inadequate living conditions, poor social support and adverse life events. A particular correlation between the lack of diverse social ties to friends, family, work and community and an increased resistance to infection has been also been identified (Cohen et al, 1997).

Individuals with a mental health problem often find themselves 'among the most unequal, disenfranchised, disempowered and excluded members' of our communities (Mentality and NIMHE 2004c). According to the Social Exclusion Unit (2004), one of the main causes of this 'cycle of exclusion' is stigma and discrimination which unfortunately still remains pervasive throughout society. The Disability Rights Commission (2006) found that people with mental health problems are more likely to be living in poverty and in socially deprived areas and are also more likely to find themselves excluded, or discriminated, against in schools, workplaces, health services and local communities.

These negative attitudes can manifest in a range of adverse material conditions, including unemployment, poverty and debt, homelessness, loss of social networks and rejection from society. It is estimated that one in four tenants with mental health problems is in rent arrears and at risk of losing their home. Fewer than 10 employers say they would recruit someone with a mental health problem, forcing individuals to depend on state benefits which can be further reduced during a period of hospitalisation. The government estimates that only 24% of adults with long term mental health problems are in work. This is the lowest employment rate for any of the main groups of disabled people. Over 900,000 adults claiming sickness and disability benefits, in England, identify mental health problems as their primary condition. Individuals with mental health problems who are in employment are at more than double the risk of losing their job than those without (Social Exclusion Unit, 2004).

Individuals often encounter barriers to engaging in the community and struggle to access facilities in education, the arts, sports and leisure, often because providers are unsure how to target their services to make them more inclusive and low expectations of what these individuals can achieve (Social Exclusion Unit, 2004).

Overcoming the Problem

The need to address such issues and improve the physical health of mental health service users, is now inescapable and has been afforded priority and is supported by service user perspectives (DH, 2006; SNMAC, 2006; Mentality and NIMHE, 2004; NICE, 2006; Disability Rights Commission, 2006; NMC, 2006). There is also increasing acknowledgment within the nursing profession that 'people with mental health problems need support from mental health nurses to ensure they have access to appropriate physical health care and regular assessment of their physical needs' (DH, 2006). Mental health professionals therefore need to develop an awareness of physical health needs and be clinically equipped to address these is essential to facilitate positive change.

What action can be taken to ensure that physical health care is high on the agenda? Stigma, discrimination and exclusion within the healthcare system have been identified as significant barriers to equal access to services and treatment.

One of the first steps, therefore, is to appreciate that service users are concerned with their physical health; contrary to stereotypical views they are interested and motivated to engage in activities to improve, and/or maintain, their physical health and would like health professionals to take this aspect of their health seriously. Once acknowledgment of this is made, opportunities for facilitating and enabling change are possible. Challenging perceptions, attitudes and beliefs is, as *Figure 1* illustrates, a cornerstone of positive change, and the more practice changes to accommodate and respond to this view, the more inclusive and less discriminatory services become. To achieve this, everyone dealing with individuals with mental health difficulties, in primary and secondary care, needs to be informed and made aware of how issues such as inequality, exclusion and discrimination could compromise a successful health care experience. Mandatory disability equality and awareness training is one recommendation made by the Disability Rights Commission to tackle the stigma associated with (learning disability and) mental health, encourage a more holistic approach and reduce the incidence of diagnostic overshadowing (Disability Rights Commission, 2006). Further recommendations include ensuring that training is evidence-based and

Figure 1. Challenging perceptions, attitudes and beliefs in mental health illness

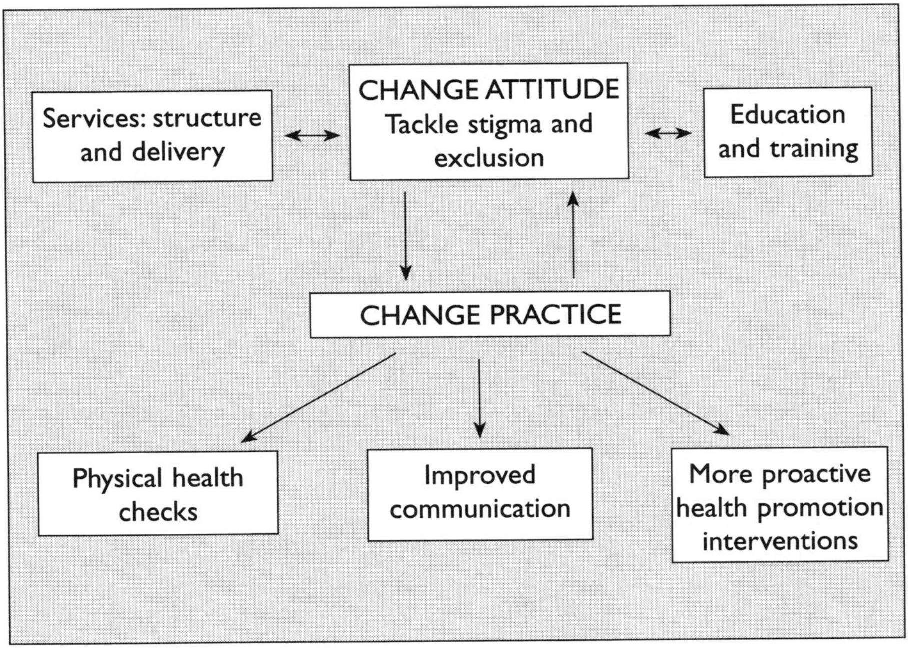

developed and delivered in consultation and collaboration with service users. It is also suggested that such training should extend to the decision makers within services to ensure service structure supports these aims.

One of the most consistent recommendations found in the literature is the need for regular physical health checks which should, at a minimum, be carried out annually (DH, 2006). It is suggested such checks should be used as an opportunity to both gather and offer information about current medication and known illness, weight (in relation to height) and BMI, lifestyle factors such as, diet, exercise, alcohol and drug use, sexual behaviour and smoking. Information about current physical symptoms should also be included as should routine monitoring of blood pressure, glucose and cholesterol levels. Preventative measures such as cervical smears, breast and prostate screening, bone density measurement and the flu' vaccination should also be considered alongside a review of other physical health needs such as dentistry, chiropody, sexually transmitted diseases, sight and hearing.

However, for any health check to be successful other factors, such as establishing clear professional roles and responsibilities and ensuring those responsible possess the requisite knowledge and skills need also to be considered.

Although the new General Medical Services (nGMS) contract (NHS, 2005) states that the physical health care of individuals with severe mental illness is the responsibility of primary care, active links and effective communication between primary and secondary are essential. This can be facilitated through regular contact and correspondence between the services. For service users cared for in the community these should occur, at a minimum, every three months. The nGMS contract also requires that a register of all individuals with a diagnosis of schizophrenia and bi-polar disorder be established in each GP practice to enable specific care, and the annual health check to be targeted at this group. Although this is limited to the more severe forms of diagnosis, at present the Disability Rights Commission (2006) suggest that this be extended to include other vulnerable groups.

It is also recommended that a physical health check should be carried out at the point of first contact to all services, admission to hospital and/or prison and on discharge. Particular attention should also be given to individuals who have limited access to GPs, such as the homeless.

Information about physical care should be clearly documented and included in care plans. Individual roles and responsibilities need also to be clearly identified and documented (DH, 2006).

Inter-professional Communication and Training

Inter-professional communication and inter-personal skills are equally essential to include and share information with the service user and carers ,if appropriate. Opportunities for service users to express themselves can be further facilitated by allowing time and flexibility.

As previously suggested, a lack of relevant training and experience can result in a situation where physical symptoms are ignored, both by mental health care professionals who are inadequately prepared to recognise and manage physical conditions, and professionals without specific mental health training (Disability Rights Commission, 2006). Provision of relevant training is, therefore, essential. This view is endorsed through the *Essential Skills Clusters* introduced by the Nursing & Midwifery Council (NMC, 2006) for implementation by September 2008 and the Chief Nursing Officers Review of Mental Health Nursing (2006), which highlights the need for mental health nurses to promote the physical health of service users and demonstrate the knowledge and competencies necessary to meet this requirement.

In terms of pre-registration nurse training, it has been suggested that programmes should ensure that physical and mental health aspects of care are more integrated and include training in basic physical and mental health assessment and therapeutic engagement across branches (Muir-Cochrane, 2006). Certainly, in the light of recent publications, institutions of Higher Education are obliged to ensure that these essential items are explicitly embedded in pre-registration curricula. It is also essential that opportunities for post-registration training should be made available to ensure that the knowledge and skills of the existing workforce is at a level appropriate to both meet the needs of its service users and support and develop the skills of more recently trained health care workers.

Whilst it is clear that education and healthcare providers need to take responsibility for providing and creating opportunities for, relevant training programmes, it is also essential that individual healthcare workers share this responsibility by recognising deficits in their knowledge, skills and experience and taking remedial action to address these. Ensuring concepts such as reflection, life-long learning, clinical supervision and personal and professional development continue to be endorsed will further facilitate this process.

Once information about physical health status is gathered, documented and disseminated, there is opportunity to offer advice, interventions and support around a range of issues such as medication management, nutrition, smoking, physical activity and stress management.

Management of Medication

Most service users will be using some prescribed medication as a method of managing psychiatric signs and symptoms, however, as previously indicated, the majority of prescribed drugs also cause unwanted and often physically damaging side effects. It is essential, therefore to ensure that medication is routinely reviewed by the prescriber, or whoever is responsible for monitoring medication, to ensure a balance between mental stability and quality of life is achieved (DH, 2006).

Again, an effective system requires good communication between professionals and the clinical skills and knowledge to perform related health checks (weight, blood pressure and any further relevant blood tests such as white cell counts, thyroid function, renal function and serum lithium levels). Accessible information, and the opportunity for further discussion, about all prescribed medication should be provided, including a list of unwanted effects so service users can make informed choices with respect to their overall health.

Increasing Activity Levels

Increasing activity levels will contribute to the prevention and management of a range of diseases including coronary heart disease, stroke, osteoporosis, diabetes and cancer, and is a useful intervention for weight management, which has beneficial effects on mental health. Exercise is consistently associated with positive mood and can also help reduce the symptoms of anxiety and non-clinical depression, help manage the positive symptoms of schizophrenia, stress, and helps promote sleep. Physical activity also has the potential to improve the quality of life for people with severe mental illness as participation in exercise can decrease social isolation, promote a sense of normalisation and offer safe opportunities for social interaction.

On this basis, and as an intervention valued by service users, it has been suggested that along with other healthy living interventions clinicians should consider physical activity as a routine aspect of care (DH, 2006).

One of the major barriers preventing the promotion of increased levels of physical activity are fears about safety, so although moderate intensity activity is relatively safe in high risk populations it is advisable to get medical clearance first. In terms of designing an achievable and sustainable activity programme it appears that adherence rates for psychiatric service users do not differ much from other population groups. However, programmes that are culturally sensitive and tailored to individual needs tend to be more effective (Richardson et al, 2005). Lifestyle interventions such as walking can provide a low-cost alternative to structured programmes, can be integrated into daily schedules and can be performed individually or as part of a group. Other factors that appear to promote adherence are avoiding unrealistic expectations, setting small incremental increases and goals, and providing supportive leadership with plenty of positive feedback and reinforcement.

Improved Diet

Changes to dietary intake can also have a beneficial effect on physical and mental health and is an important aspect of weight management (Mental Health Foundation, 2006; Sustain, 2006). General dietary advice which helps maintain a healthy body weight and contribute to the prevention and management of diseases such as cardiovascular disease, diabetes, cancer and obesity, includes eating five or more portions of fruit and vegetables per day, reducing intakes of, particularly, saturated fats, reducing salt intake and eating at least two portions of fish, one of which should be oily, per week (British Nutrition Foundation, 2007).

Although there are obvious barriers to achieving this in a population group which is socio-economically challenged, positive changes can still be accomplished and are welcomed by service users. Organisations such as Rethink and the Mental Health Foundation also provide information on how to achieve a balanced diet with limited finances and resources.

Lifestyle groups can be a useful method of sharing information and experiences and can contribute to positive changes in lifestyle with regards to diet, physical activity and smoking cessation (DH, 2006; Law, 2007). Further benefits include increases in social inclusion and self esteem.

Effective inter-professional working is, again, essential and can be further facilitated by including dieticians and nutritionists within the team. Keeping up-to-date with current available evidence and examples of good practice, which can be adapted for implementation in a variety of care settings, is also a way of developing practice and improving health outcomes.

Smoking Cessation

NICE (2006) Guidelines recommend that all people who smoke should be asked how interested they are in stopping. Although this may not be appropriate at times when symptoms are at their most active, this should not prevent subsequent interventions as, although there is evidence of less success in this population group than in the general population, there is still a significant success rate (Bradshaw et al, 2005b). Smoking cessation guidelines for health workers recommend the 'four A's' approach:

- Ask
- Advise
- Assist
- Arrange.

With regards to specific interventions, it appears that a combination of approaches, such as individual and/or group therapy, with nicotine replacement therapy has a better long term outcome than a singular approach and/or brief opportunistic advice (Bradshaw, 2005b).

Abstinence rates also appear higher in individuals who are prescribed atypical anti-psychotics, and because of the effects tobacco can have on antipsychotic medication a review of medication is advisable.

Learning Points

1. Individuals with a mental health diagnosis have higher rates of physical illness resulting in increased morbidity and mortality
2. A combination of lifestyle, treatment and socio-economic factors are instrumental in this process
3. Contrary to stereotypical views, service users are interested in their physical health and want health professionals to take this aspect of their health seriously
4. Good physical health is a realistic goal for mental health service users
5. Measures to promote, maintain and improve the physical health of mental health service users are possible.

Resources

Rethink: www.rethink.org.uk

Mental Health Foundation: www.mentalhealth.org.uk

References

Baxter D (1996) The Mortality Experience of Individuals on the Salford Psychiatric Case register: All cause mortality. *British Journal of Psychiatry* 168: 772-779

Blows W (2003) *The Biological Basis of Nursing: Mental Health*. Routledge, London

Bradshaw T, Lovell K, Harris N (2005) Healthy Living Interventions with Schizophrenia: a systematic review. *Journal of Advanced Nursing* **49**(6): 634-654

British Nutrition Foundation (2007) *Heart Disease and Stroke*. British Nutrition Foundation, London

Brown S, Inskip H, Barraclough B (2000) Causes of the excess mortality of schizophrenia. *British Journal of Psychiatry* **177**: 212-217

Brown S, Birtwistle J, Roe L, Thompson C (1999) The unhealthy lifestyle of people with schizophrenia. *Psychological Medicine* **29**: 697-701

Cohen A, Hove M (2001) *Physical Health of People with Severe Mental Illness: a training pack for GP Educators.* The Sainsbury Centre for Mental Health, London

Cohen S, Kessler R, Underwood Gordon L (1995) *Measuring Stress: A guide for health and social scientists.* Oxford University Press, Oxford

Cohen S, Doyle W, Skoner D, Rabin B, Gwaltney J (1997) Social ties and susceptibility to the common cold. *JAMA* **277**(24): 1940-1944

Dean J, Todd G, Morrow H, Sheldon K (2001) Mum, I used to be good looking but look at me now: the physical health needs of adults with mental health problems. The Perspectives of Users, Carers and Front-Line Staff. *International Journal of Mental Health Promotion* **3**(4): 16-24

DH (2006) *Choosing Health: Supporting the Needs of People with Severe Mental Illness: Commissioning Framework.* Department of Health, London

DH (2006) *Self-Assessment Toolkit. From Values to Action: The Chief Nursing Officer's Review of Mental Health Nursing.* Department of Health, London

DH (2006) *Best Practice Competencies and Capabilities for Pre-registration Mental Health Nurses in England: The Chief Nursing Officer's Review of Mental Health Nursing.* Department of Health, London

DH (2006) *Chief Nursing Officer's Review of Mental Health Nursing: Summary of Responses to the Consultation.* Department of Health, London

DH (2005) *Meeting the Physical Needs of Individuals with Mental Health Problems and the Mental Health Needs of Individuals.* Department of Health, London

DH (2005) *Choosing Activity.* Department of Health, London

DH (1999) *A National Service Framework for Mental Health.* Department of Health, London

DH (1992) *The Health of the Nation.* Department of Health, London

Dickinson A, Welch C, Ager L, Costar A (2005) Hospital Mealtimes: action research for Change. *Proceedings of the Nutrition Society* **64**: 269-275

Disability Rights Commission (2006) *Equal Treatment: Closing the Gap. A formal investigation into physical health inequalities experienced by people with learning disabilities and/or mental health Stratford upon Avon.* Disability Rights Commission, London

Faulkner G (2005) Exercise as an Adjunct Treatment for Schizophrenia. In: Faulkner, G, Taylor A, eds. *Exercise, Health and Mental Health: Emerging relationships.* Routledge, Abingdon

Forrest E (2006) Body of evidence. *Health Service Journal* **23**: 23-26

Goldman, L. (1999) Medical illness in patients with schizophrenia. *Journal of Clinical Psychiatry* **60**(21): 10-15

Jeste D, Gladsjo J, Lindamer L, Lacro J (1996) Medical co-morbidity in schizophrenia. *Schizophrenia Bulletin* **22**: 413-427

Kendrick T (1995) Randomised controlled trial of teaching general practitioners to carry out structured assessments of their long-term mentally ill patients. *British Medical Journal* **311**: 93-98

Law D (2007) Physical health: how to minimise the risks faced by patients with schizophrenia. *Mental Health Practice March* **10**(6): 26-28

Le Fevre PD (2001) Improving the physical health of patients with schizophrenia: therapeutic nihilism or realism? *Scottish Medical Journal* **46**: 011-013

Marder S (2004) Physical health monitoring of patients with schizophrenia. *American Journal of Psychiatry* **61**(8): 334-1349

McCreadie R (2002) Use of drugs, alcohol and tobacco by people with schizophrenia: case control study. *British Journal of Psychiatry* **181**(4): 321-325

Meaney AM, Smith S, Howes OD, O'Brien M, Murray RM, O'Keane V (2004) Effects of long-term prolactin-raising antipsychotic medication on bone mineral density in patients with schizophrenia. *British Journal of Psychiatry* **184**: 503-508

Mental Health Foundation (2005) *Up and Running.* Mental Health Foundation, London

Mental Health Foundation (2006) *Feeding Minds: The Impact of Food on Mental Health.* Mental Health Foundation, London

Mentality and NIHME (2004a) *Healthy Body and Mind: promoting healthy living for people who experience mental distress: A guide for people working in community mental health services.* Mentality and NIHME

Mentality and NIHME (2004b) *Healthy Body and Mind: promoting healthy living for people who experience mental distress: A guide for people working in inpatient services.* Mentality and NIHME

Mentality and NIHME (2004c) *Healthy Body and Mind: promoting healthy living for people who experience mental distress: A guide for people working in primary health care teams supporting people working with severe and enduring mental illness.* Mentality and NIHME

Mir S, Taylor D (2001) Atypical antipsychotics and hyperglycemia. *International Clinical Psychopharmacology* **16**(2): 63-73

Muir-Cochrane E (2006) Medical co-morbidity risk factors and barriers to care for people with schizophrenia. *Journal of Psychiatric and Mental Health Nursing* **13**: 447-452

NICE (2006) *Bipolar Disorder: The management of bipolar disorder in adults, children and adolescents in primary and secondary care.* NICE, London

NICE (2006) *Brief Interventions and Referral for Smoking Cessation in Primary Care and Other Settings.* NICE, London

NICE (2002) *Schizophrenia: Core Interventions in the Treatment and Management of Schizophrenia in Primary and Secondary Care*. NICE, London

National Schizophrenia Fellowship (2001) *Doesn't it Make you Sick? Side effects of medicine and physical health concerns of people with severe mental illness*. NSF, London

NHS Employers (2005) I*nvesting in General Practice: Revisions to the General Medical Service Contract for 2006-7 in England. Stage 1*. NHS Employers, London

NMC (2006) *Advance Information regarding essential Skills Clusters for Pre-Registration Nursing programmes. NMC Circular 35/2006*. NMC, London

NMC (2007) *Essential Skills Clusters for Pre-Registration Nursing Programmes*. NMC Circular 07/2007. NMC, London

Phelan M, Stradins L, Morrison S (2001) Physical Health of People with Severe Mental Illness: can be improved if primary care and mental health professionals pay attention to it. *British Medical Journal* **322**: 43-444

Phelan M, Stradins L, Amin D, Isadore R, Hitrov C, Doyle A, Inglis R (2004) The physical health check: a tool for mental health workers. *Journal of Mental Health* **13**(3): 277-284

Pulzer M (2006) Metabolic syndrome and anti-psychotic drugs. *Mental Health Nursing* **26**(6): 17-19

Rethink (2003) *Just One Per Cent: The experiences of people using mental health services*. Rethink, London

Rethink (2003) *Self-Management: the experiences and views of self management of people with a diagnosis of schizophrenia*. Rethink, London

Rethink (2003) *Smoking and Mental Illness*. Rething, London

Roberts L, et al (2007) Physical health care of patients with schizophrenia in primary care: a comparative study. *Family Practice: An International Journal* **24**(1): 34-40

Robson D, Gray R (2005) Can we help people with schizophrenia stop smoking? *Mental Health Practice* **9**(4): 15-18

Social Exclusion Unit (2004) *Mental Health and Social Exclusion*. Office of the Deputy Prime Minister, London

Stahl S (2000) *Essential Psychopharmacology: Neuroscientific basis and practical applications*. 2nd edn. Cambridge University Press

Sustain (2006) *Changing Diets, Changing Minds: How food affects mental well being and behaviour*. Sustain Publications, London

Usher K, Foster K, Park T (2006) The metabolic syndrome and schizophrenia: the latest evidence and nursing guidelines for management. *Journal of Psychiatric and Mental Health Nursing* **13**: 730-734

CHAPTER 12

Common Mental Health Problems in Primary Care

Dave Kingdon

This chapter orientates the reader to the nature and context of primary care mental health, introducing some recent features of Department of Health planning and guidance in the field of psychological therapies for common mental health problems. It also provides a counter discourse to the dominant paradigm in psychological therapies evidence and visits the therapeutic relationship, which is viewed as the social and dynamic milieu in which beneficial understanding, insights and learning can occur. In doing so, key psychodynamic and relational principles are highlighted within this context, and case studies are provided to assist the reader in theoretical case conceptualisation.

Psychological Interventions and the Nature of Common Mental Health Problems in Primary Care Settings

The report highlighting the economic burden of depressive illnesses by Richard Layard in 2005 has done much to raise the profile of common mental health problems within the health community, policy makers and commissioners. It has also highlighted the lack in provision of psychological treatments available, their patchy provision and limited accessibility. Following on, the National Institute for Mental Health and Care Services in Partnership have sought to address this through a number of initiatives under the heading of Improving Access to Psychological Therapies. As a result, a small number of pilot sites have been developed with this agenda.

According to Layard's (2005) findings there are more mentally ill people receiving incapacity benefits than the total number of unemployed people on benefit, and that one in six of all people suffer from depression or chronic anxiety, which affects one in three of all families. He continues to report that only a quarter of those who are ill are receiving any treatment — in most cases medication, and that modern evidence-based psychological therapy is as effective as medication and is preferred by the majority of patients.

In reviewing the evidence for psychological therapies, Layard naturally found more support for cognitive behavioural therapy than other therapies. This is due to the fact the cognitive behavioural approach lends itself to the scientific and positivist research paradigm and is predominantly the approach used and researched by clinical psychologists. Scepticism and concern, however, is raised by many other schools of psychological therapy for its reductionistic methods and their inherent inadequacies within the field of psychological therapies (Holmes, 2002; Marzillier, 2004; Goldbeck-Wood and Fonagy, 2004). That said; it has provided a platform for Layard to project the financial viability of a course of up to 20 therapy sessions to help an individual to rejoin society through return to work, would pay for itself in money saved on incapacity benefits and lost tax receipts. Within this context, the introduction of more psychological therapists into the NHS is welcomed.

Dovetailing with recent guidance from NICE (2004) in the treatment and management of Depression, *Generalised Anxiety and Post Traumatic Stress Disorder*, the psychological approaches generally recommended continue to fall within the cognitive behavioural paradigm (DH, 2001). Further, the Stepped Care model (Paxton et al, 2000) has been developed as a way of adhering to this evidence, and attempting to 'provide significant health gain' and 'derive greatest benefits from available therapeutic resources' (Bower and Gilbody, 2005). This has been implemented in a variety of ways, for example at the Doncaster pilot site, where services are structured in this way, which means that referrals are triaged and subsequently allocated to the most appropriate resource, including telephone consultancy (DH, 2007; Gray, 2007).

The Common Mental Health Problem Service (CMHPS), Leicestershire, was part commissioned in 2001 as a prompt response to the National Service Framework, following consultation with User groups, GPs and PCT leads (DH, 1999). As such, large funding was secured and Leicestershire progressed beyond some of the guidance, which later emerged from NIMHE and the Department of Health (DH, 2003; NICE, 2004; NIMHE, 2004). As a result, the CMHPS adopted a robust and comprehensive model, employing skilled therapists with both experience in statutory mental health work, as well as post registration training within a psychological model (psychodynamic, cognitive behavioural, interpersonal psychotherapy, cognitive analytic therapy). The CMHPS received strong support following an audit into primary care services provision by the Sainsbury Centre for Mental Health (Durcan and Knowles, 2004). In doing so, practitioners recruited were qualified to manage and treat a wide range of clinical complaints successfully.

Whilst recognising the strategy involved and applied within the stepped care model and NICE guidelines, in practice a wide range of factors cannot always be strategically managed in this way. For example, there are variety of co-morbid conditions including mixed anxiety and depressive states, severe stress reactions and burn out, alcohol and drug problems, domestic violence and relationship issues, adjustments, suicidal states and long-standing underlying trauma including childhood sexual abuse. From this point of view simple presentations of anxiety, phobia and depression are less workable diagnosis in routine practice, and thus the implementation of standardised treatment packages, manuals or computerised cognitive behavioural therapy are challenged (Craig and Boardman,1997; Niles et al, 2005).

Through service audit and evaluation the CMHPS received approximately 33000 referrals over a 2-year period, with high levels of distress as measured by the CORE outcome measure (Evans et al, 2002). This revealed over 50% of referrals experiencing moderate-severe and severe symptomology. This is comparable with the level of distress referred to psychiatric teams elsewhere in the country (Gilbert, 2005). Furthermore, our records showed that over 50% of these referrals were managing to continue working, with around 20% either receiving incapacity benefit or on sick leave due to their mental health problems.

Primary Care: The Clinical Setting

The primary care setting, notably the GP surgery, is familiar to us all. Because this is such a well-known setting, all sorts of associations, both good and bad are often attributed. This may be due to previous experiences of hospitals, doctors and healthcare professionals, individual successes or failures in health treatments, and through earlier experiences of being ill. Overall, local access and a level of public confidence in the medical setting is seen as a strength in accessing health support and was behind some of the plans held within the National Service Framework standard 2 (DH, 1999).

The first observation is that surgeries always appear busy and that there are many competing demands on the time of receptionists, nurses, health visitors and GPs. Furthermore, a wide variety of complaints are assessed, triaged, treated and managed within this setting and we can see parallels of this within mental health. Primary care is seen as the 'gateway' into any NHS treatments and as such most health and social needs are brought into this setting.

Petrioni (1995) describes how practitioners need to be generalist specialists, carrying a broad working knowledge of a range of conditions and presentations. Furthermore, Weiner et al (1988) describes the notion of the Arab 'souk' or market place, where everything is on offer and equally in demand. From this point of view, mental health workers in GP surgeries may receive referrals for a wide range of complaints.

The key facility in providing the model of 'in-house' psychological therapist means that a patient who is at any stage of their condition may seek a consultation. I will explore this further from the psychodynamic perspective below, as we note that people use consultations in many different ways. The skilled therapist is sufficiently confident to tune into the patients' need as well as considering their level of readiness or commitment to change (Prochaska and Di Clemente, 1982).

Work is currently in progress to identify and develop key competencies within mental health therapies (DH, 2007). It is the contention of the author, that as well as Cognitive Behavioural and Problem solving skills, therapists are also cognisant of the fundamentals of developmental and psychodynamic psychology (see also Perris, 2005).

Observations on Key Psychodynamic Themes

We cannot introduce psychodynamic theory without emphasising the importance of the therapeutic relationship as the main vehicle for therapeutic change. Whilst this has been inherently recognised within psychodynamic traditions, it is now becoming accepted as significant across all therapies including cognitive behavioural therapies (Lewis, 2000; Catty, 2005; Gilbert, 2006).

It is now becoming widely acknowledged that all relationships carry some form of transference, counter transference and projective identification (Gilbert 2006, Andersen and Baum 1994, Luborsky 1997). As such, the reenactments evident and often most pronounced during initial clinical encounters can be most telling. I will return to this with the case studies later in the chapter.

Psychotherapeutic interventions can be seen as processes of relationship building, as well as offering remedial and facilitative opportunities. Generally, psychodynamic theory (in which I will include child development and object relations theories), provide a useful therapeutic framework which the therapist can operate from. These are fairly well known and briefly outlined as follows.

The 'Good Enough Mother'

Winnicott (1960) termed the phrase the 'good enough mother' for those who manage the needs and frustrations of their baby without offering too much, nor too little. Features in children such as 'frustration tolerance' are seen as healthy, whilst 'instant gratification' suggests a frailty in the parent to withstand a struggle and can lead to later difficulties for both parties.

Attunement is regarded as an essential quality of good parenting (Ainsworth, 1985; Bowlby, 1979) whilst withholding, reticence, or withdrawal by the mother can lead the child to the limit or hide their true feelings. Optimum conditions, as in the 'good enough' which the mother strives to provide, lead to a healthy position for emotional and physical development.

Increasing findings in neuropsychiatry are now able to support the biological effects of maternal deprivation. It is interesting that Bowlby's observations on this social phenomena are now able to be recognised through physical and psychobiological development (Perry et al, 1995; Teicher et al, 2003; Schore, 2001).

Emotional Holding and Containing

'Psychotherapeutic holding' refers to the management of space of separation between infant and mother (Winnicott, 1960). It is the mother's role (or primary carer) to protect this and be sensitive to its management.

The 'containing' role of the mother provides nurturing and acceptance, so that when the child experiences natural impulses and responds with tears, anger and other emotions such as joy, that she (or the primary carer) will be comfortable enough within herself to bear the majority of such expressions without shaming, judging or criticising the child. When this happens to a satisfactory level, the infant can develop with confidence and a healthy view of themselves and others within their world.

Recent work in regard to mental health promotion now highlights emotional resilience as a key factor in maintaining a mental health balance even in the face of adversity.

Ego Defence Mechanisms / Defensive Adaptations

When 'good enough' parenting fails to occur (for whatever reason), the child experiencing natural growth pains (such as frustration, rebelliousness and other identity needs) is forced to adapt their authentic expressions, adopting a number of commonly recognised distortions known as ego defense mechanisms (Freud, 1968). These include

- Denial — (*'It is not really happening'*)
- Repression — (*'It never happened'*)
- Dissociation — (*'I do not remember what happened'*)
- Projection — (*'It is happening to you, not me'*)
- Conversion — (*'I eat and have sex when I feel it happening'*)
- Minimizing — (*'It happened but it is no big deal'*).

We might all identify with some of these adaptations, especially when we experience shock or high emotional states, however, in their extreme forms, such traits can lead to features such as addictive behaviours, eating disorders, antisocial activities and suicidal states. Maintaining such adaptations can also be seen to lead to what has been termed a 'false self' (Winnicott, 1960; Horney, 1945).

It is clear to see the importance of early emotional attachment and the attachment figure in setting up a blueprint for healthy striving and growth (both physically and mentally) to occur. The mother and father play a considerable role in this process, whether they are cohabiting or absent (or both).

Factors such as the wider family, its culture and attitude, add to the emotional chemistry and social adaptation that underlies what we broadly consider to be personality. Each of these, at differing stages, will add to the 'container' originally holding the child, namely the mother. If this is well nourished and is in itself able to express and receive love and respect, then core climate is established.

Of course, the random nature of the human experience will present its challenge to even the most robust of soils. When sudden tragedy occurs leaving families stranded and torn by whatever has befallen them, the impact of some events play their part trans-generationally. When this happens, severe adaptation is forced upon the child, and in effect, human beings do the best that they can, with the resources that they have in order to survive.

Clinical Findings and Therapeutic Application

Vignettes

Three vignettes are provided to illustrate the diverse nature of mental health complaints presenting in the primary care setting, and for subsequent consideration. Identifiable features of the cases have been altered and fictionalised to preserve anonymity, but aim to retain some of the characteristics of routine presentations in the primary care setting. At this stage, I would invite the reader to reflect on each vignette and begin to consider what type of therapeutic climate and style may need to be adopted to assist. For each case, try to identify three further components:

1.   What have been the key characteristics of episode leading up to coming for help?
2.   What were the key characteristics of the earlier emotional injuries?
3.   What do you notice about the way the patient relates to the therapist?

Vignette I

A professional woman in her late 20s attended with problems noted as low self-esteem. On examination she described a two-year relationship with an older man. She reported how he had become jealous of her attention from other men whilst she was at work, and since then had undermined her, begun to suggest what she should and should not wear, become irritable and moody whenever she displayed any autonomy in her life. To this extent she stopped wearing make up, dressed down and had stopped meeting her friends. On further questioning it became apparent that he had been violent towards her on three occasions and she agreed with me that at times she had felt manipulated into having sex with him. They did not live together.

At the initial session I put back to her that her self-esteem appeared to be affected by this highly controlling relationship which undermined her freedoms in all sorts of ways. I also pointed out the profile of abusive characters and suggested she might find support via the local domestic violence network. She said she was grateful for the time to talk, and that it had confirmed her thoughts, as indeed many friends had pointed out to her. We agreed to meet three weeks later to see what had changed and to establish any further help she may need.

On reflection of this first session, I felt satisfied that this bright and professionally successful woman could become free of this ogreous man once and for all, and begin to live a satisfying life. I was pleased to have drawn out some of his characteristics, sufficient to recognise him as potentially aggressive and dangerous to her; both to warn and inform her of his personality, and to help her to comprehend the risks involved with trying to break free. (Domestic violence claims the lives of two women every week in the UK and accounts for 16% of crime according to the Home Office.)

When she returned, I was surprised to quickly learn that she had not taken any action along the aforementioned lines, and that despite discussing attending *Relate* together [a counselling service], there was no change in the relationship status. Once again there had been arguments, coerced sex and again an incident of violence.

I was drawn to wonder what kept her in the relationship. She mentioned that her partner was going through some family stress having lost his mother, and she seemed to be displaying some strong caring and rescuing motives. She went on to say that this was the third relationship where there had been domestic violence.

On further examination, I was able to elicit that when she was growing up her father began to display some critical and erratic behaviour, which undermined her self-esteem and caused her shame and humiliation.

Vignette 2

Another referral which came my way involved a woman in her mid 30s who was experiencing persistent low mood, tearfulness, apathy, she had fleeting suicidal ideas and wanted to run away from her responsibilities as a mother to her 3-year-old daughter. There was some indication that post natal depression had been diagnosed after the birth of her daughter. She felt a failure, hopeless about recovery and was frightened. Two years previously, her father had died following a terminal illness, which had involved her frequently visiting him in the hospital some 40 miles away over a 12-month period. She had taken sick leave for the past seven weeks and could not bear to face returning to work at her part-time job. She stopped going out socially and was uncommunicative at home with her husband.

After our initial meeting, she expressed frustration and despair at having to wait for three weeks before we could meet again.

During the second interview, I was able to enquire about her general upbringing and earlier influences in her family. At this point she began to talk about how she had a congenital problem for which she received a number of operations when she was a child. This meant that she had to spend long periods in hospital between the ages of 5–10 years-old. She went on to say how she had not really thought about these aspects of her childhood until now, although there had been some discussion about the hereditary incidence of this condition when her daughter was born, although it was quickly determined that she was not affected.

As she explored her memories further, she remembered long periods of isolation at the hospital, her parents visiting and bringing grapes; feeling very awkward because they had to drive along way to get there. In particular she remembered not receiving any visit at all on her 8th birthday. In the session she was in touch with deep sadness and was tearful as she felt some of the pain and emotional agony that had gone through.

Vignette 3

Robert had been seen by a psychiatrist twice in the year before he came to see me. He felt that he had been misunderstood and found the experience unhelpful. Despite intense suicidal feelings, depressive symptoms, features of dissociation and anger, he was unhappy with the conversations at the outpatient department and was uncomfortable with the medication he was offered, which left him feeling drowsy and numb. He attended an initial assessment session with me, and despite offering to meet with him in the near future, he failed to return until finally booking himself in six months later. He was in his early 20s and had taken medical discharge from the navy where he had been training and serving for three years, and displayed some suicidal behaviour.

He was softly spoken, articulate, and slight of build. He presented with a full house of depressive symptoms including frequent suicidal fantasies of hanging himself with a rope from the garage — his only deterrent being that his younger brother might be the one to find him. He was socially isolated and showed features of social anxiety. He was trying, unsuccessfully, to find employment and felt humiliated by attending the job centre.

As we continued to meet once a fortnight he began to reveal a tragic story of persistent social bullying and emotional abuse throughout his childhood. As the son of the chairman of a highly successful international business, Robert's family moved abroad when he was nine years old until the age of 15. He was sent to a school accommodating overseas pupils, which also became his social community. He gradually revealed episodes of humiliation, victimisation and physical assaults. Much of this he kept quiet about, and when he did try talking to his parents or teachers, he was dismissed, disbelieved and discounted. When he made the transition back to Britain, he struggled to integrate to an already established school peer group and his isolation was intensified.

He recognised his desire to join the armed forces as an attempt to build his physical strength, confidence and self-esteem; however as someone with a slight build and shy demeanour he was once again an easy target. He told me about shaming and deeply humiliating episodes by his peers as well as ongoing bullying and abuse.

Since returning to live with his parents he had established contact with some remaining school friends, although felt very emotionally distant and disconnected from them, struggling with trust and openness. His role had become that of the clown, or joker, and in this sense he had become popular, however he was now becoming aware of playing an inauthentic role, which was masking some of his deeper fears. He tried using alcohol to help him maintain this façade, but found that this resulted in dramatic mood swings, including anger outbursts.

Discussion

These three vignettes highlight the diversity of clinical presentations within primary care, and also demonstrate that therapists need to be able to manage such diversity with confidence. Each case represents difficulties at the Stepped Care Level 3 or above, with moderate to severe symptomology. Whilst we might consider that each of the cases qualifies with a diagnosis of clinical depression, we can also see that these cases are more complex.

Malan (1979) and Luborsky (1984, 1997) amongst others, have demonstrated how core psychological conflicts become central to the individuals ways of relating and being. Along these lines, therapists attempt to identify key characteristics of early patterns of relating with significant others and subsequently to a broader world in the 'here and now'. Specific attention is also drawn to the way the patient relates to the therapist; once again to support and confirm the texture of these patterns.

It is also interesting to note the studies reported by Miranda and Anderson (2007) which demonstrate how individuals respond rapidly to transference cues at an emotional level. Recent studies in behavioural and social cognitions are, therefore showing clearly what occurs between individuals and what is heightened within the therapeutic situation and relationship.

It is through the provision of the safe and secure base, and the steady provision of a therapeutic relationship, that both understandings and the beginnings of new ways of relating can be developed. As Guntrip (1975) has noted of this process:

> *'...the provision of a reliable and understanding human relationship, of a kind that makes contact with the deeply repressed traumatized child in a way that enables the patient to become steadily more able to live in the security of a new real relationship, with the traumatic legacy of the earliest formative years, as it seeps through, or erupts into consciousness'*
>
> *Guntrip, 1975*

In the three vignettes highlighted, we can see that each of them are likely to require special attention in regard to 'how' the therapist behaves.

In the first case, it appears that a possible struggle is about to emerge between us, as we are all drawn into attempting to rescue the other, whilst losing site of our own responsibilities and limits. This would be the injury that she may have suffered when her father became 'ill' and erratic in his behaviour, causing her deep humiliation, which she could only bear by seeing her father as needing help.

In the second case, the therapeutic relationship was quickly called into question when the initial gap in setting up appointments immediately created a form of abandonment.

In the third case, steady processes of trust building and sensitivity with validation would appear to be part of the ingredients required to begin to overcome the tender wounds just beneath the surface.

No doubt in each case some rupture may emerge and the therapist may find themselves letting the patient down. Furthermore, the patterns of adaptation which the patient has learnt may also in turn cause the therapist to 'play into the script'. Thus, as Bowlby (1979) highlights:

> *'...we find each patient confined within a more or less closed system and only slowly, often inch by inch, is it possible for him to escape'*
>
> *Bowlby, 1979*

Certainly, within the primary care provision of psychological therapies, intensive psychotherapy is unviable to sustain. As a result, consideration as to the patient's capacity to manage transference interpretations is important. None the less, inquiry regarding the quality of 'out there' interpersonal relationships and building on their qualities, whilst watching out for distorted re-enactments can be facilitative and helpful.

Returning to the vignettes once more, vignette 1 attended for a series of seven sessions. She became more upset at the actions of her father when she was a teenager, but also began to understand that he had been under significant pressures, which she later found out about. This helped her to realise that it was not herself who had done anything wrong. This released both her guilt and anger, as well as helping her to see that her rescuing attempts were misguided. She also realised how this pattern of relating to men had developed. Eventually, she decided to leave her partner when he showed no commitment to attend a *Relate* session, and fortunately there were no violent repercussions.

Vignette2, only attended for one further session. She had set up a self help/awareness group for people suffering with the condition she had as a child. She felt energised by this and presented with a rapid remission of symptoms. She felt closer to her child and also her mother, as she now had understood where her anger and feelings of loss had come from. There was a texture here of 'flight into health' and I was surprised when she said she felt well enough to continue without further help. A key benefit of the 'in-house' therapist is the facility to see someone again swiftly and easily without a lengthy referral process. In this case a process of 'watchful waiting (see Stepped Care model) can be achieved.

Vignette 3 became a more protracted treatment, which involved continuous attempts to maintain reliability, consistency and a place to provide validation and authenticity. Trust and humiliation were central themes, and as a secure base was provided, the patient was gradually able to explore his wider milieu. He told many stories of his tragic experiences and was gradually able to express a wide range of associated emotions. This helped him to manage day-to-day emotions and learned not to overreact to negative experiences such as the job centre or aggressive looking people whilst out and about. Over the course of a year of regular meetings, Robert managed to find work with a youth charity, helping youngsters with outward-bound skills. He was gradually able to use his sensitivity to support young people, as well as begin to relate to his peers and his bosses without feeling threatened.

Common Mental Health, Skilled Therapeutic Interventions and Evidence-based Practice

The risks of neglecting clinical presentations in the primary care setting or providing ineffective treatments is potentially costly to society as a whole, both financially and emotionally; the latter in the form of family breakdown, domestic violence, depression and addictive problems, as well as neglect within the family and limited options for meaningful employment and occupation which is important not just financially but for identity and self-esteem.

Whilst there is a renewed interest in treating common mental health problems, the evidence-based literature and applied research and treatment paradigm could potentially be misleading and less effectual than expected across large populations. For example, when we examine the rapid rise and profile of computerised Cognitive Behavioural Therapy, it is interesting that a sample of 502 patients was assessed and only 274 commenced the trial (Proudfoot, 2004). With only half of this population entering the treatment group, hard findings might be difficult to assert, yet have found their way into the NICE guidelines for anxiety.

Further, fascinating commentary on the workings of NICE are also noted by Milewa and Barry (2005), who describe a range of influences which go beyond clinical and cost-effectiveness findings, and where human agency and influence can shape the nature of evidence which is proposed. On reviewing the components of the analysis which made up NICE guidelines, it is notable that whilst there are many references to randomized control trial studies and other controlled studies, they do not all measure the same features and the settings and range of interventions vary widely. Some of these comments include reference to the bias of drug companies' findings, differences in severity of patients selected for various trials, and the genuine desire for publications to wish to show positive findings rather than negative ones (NICE, 2004). As a result transferability of studies results are highly questionable when it comes to developing policy. Qualitative and subjectivist research approaches such as hermeneutics, ethnography and phenomenology however, as well as objective appraisal of positivist research studies may lead to greater understanding of some of the honest texture present within real world clinical practice.

Developing core competencies within psychotherapeutic work is seen as essential for commissioners, service planners and the public to be confident in its work force. The burgeoning rise in self-help texts, manualised treatments and protocols may be one way of learning, however, as we have seen within the case studies, only a small minority of patients presenting may benefit from these alone. The remainder appear to present with long term co-morbid conditions, frequently with underlying trauma, neglect, shame and humiliation and which will require a range of advanced practitioners to assist.

Training in psychological approaches is certainly desirable for any mental health practitioner in the majority of settings. Perris (2003) argues that therapists working in non-specialised departments should have a good training within one core model, for example cognitive behavioural therapy/analytic, but also be sufficiently competent in an alternative approach to allow for flexibility not only in treatment planning, but also to assist in case conceptualisation.

Being willing and interested to engage with patients and service users at a real, transparent and open level is a demanding task, and it is easy to see how institutional structures or even treatment manuals can provide sanctuary for anyone searching for an easier professional life. Furthermore, when therapists, first line and other helping professionals do become involved, it is important that they are adequately supported with group or individual supervision, that they stay aware of their reactions and responses, and particularly in order to ensure they refrain from acting out their own unmet needs with patients.

Working within 'managed' psychological services may be one way to mitigate against the dangers of becoming a lone practitioner, and is something that commissioners of services should value (DH, 2004). Receiving peer support, access to expert opinion, personal therapy or at least an opportunity to debrief material which a practitioner has been exposed to is our own profession responsibility to ensure that we don't become overwhelmed by mental health work. When practitioners do feel supported and valued, they may well advance to provide meaningful engagement with those in need and gradually begin to achieve real results in treatment.

Learning Points

1. Training in psychological approaches is certainly desirable for any mental health practitioner in the majority of settings
2. Working within 'managed' psychological services may be one way to mitigate against the dangers of becoming a lone practitioner, and is something that commissioners of services should value
3. Developing core competencies within psychotherapeutic work is seen as essential for commissioners, service planners and the public to be confident in its work force
4. Increasing findings in neuropsychiatry are now able to support the biological effects of maternal deprivation.

References

Andersen S, Baum A (1994) Transference in Interpersonal Relations: Inferences and Affect Based on Significant-Other Representations. *Journal of Personality* **62**(4): 459–97

Ainsworth M (1985) Patterns of infant-mother attachments: antecedents and effects on development. *Bulletin of the New York Academy of Medicine* **66**(9): 771–90

Ainsworth M, Blehar M, Waters E, Wall S (1978) *Patterns of attachment: a psychological study of the strange situation*. Lawrence Erlbraum, Hillsdale NJ

Bowlby J (1979) *The making and breaking of affectional bonds*. Tavistock, Routledge

Bowlby J (1973) Attachment and Loss. *Separation* **2:** Hogarth Press, London

Bower P, Gilbody S (2005) Stepped care in psychological therapies: access, effectiveness and efficiency. *British Journal of Psychiatry* **186:** 11–17

Bower P, Sibbald B (2000) Systematic review of the effect of on-site mental health professionals on the clinical behaviour of general practitioners. *British Medical Journal* **320:** 614–7

Catty J (2004) The Vehicle of success: Theoretical and empirical perspectives on the therapeutic alliance in psychotherapy and psychiatry. *Psychology and Psychotherapy: Theory, Research and Practice* **77:** 255–72

Craig T, Boardman A (1997) ABC of mental health: Common mental health problems in primary care. *British Medical Journal* **314:** 1609

DH (2001) *Treatment choice in psychological therapies and counselling. Evidence based practice guideline*. HMSO, London

DH (2004) *Organizing and Delivering Psychological Therapies*. HMSO, London

DH (1999) *National Service Framework*. HMSO, London

DH (1996) *NHS Psychotherapy Services in England*. DOH, London

DH (2003) *Fast Forwarding Primary Care Mental Health. Graduate Mental Health Workers. Best Practice Guidance*. HMSO, London

DH (2007) *Improving Access for Psychological Therapies*. DH publications

Durcan G, Knowles K (2004) *Audit of primary mental health care in Leicester, Leicestershire and Rutland*. Sainsbury Center for Mental Health

Evans C, Connell J, Barkham M, Margison F, Mellor-Clark J, McGrath G et al (2002) Towards a standardised brief outcome measure: psychometric properties and utilisation of the CORE-OM. *British Journal of Psychiatry* **180:** 51–60

Freud A (1968) *The Ego and Mechanisms of Defense*. Hogarth press, London

Gilbert P, Allan S, Nicholls W, Olsen K (2005) The Assessment of Psychological Symptoms of Patients Referred to Community Mental Health Teams: Distress, Chronicity and Life Interference. *Clinical Psychology and Psychotherapy Clinical Psychology and Psychotherapy* **12:** 10–27

Gilbody S (2005) Stepped care in psychological therapies: access, effectiveness and efficiency. *British Journal of Psychiatry* **186:** 11–17

Goldbeck-Wood S, Fonagy P (2004) The future of psychotherapy in the NHS. *British Medical Journal* **329:** 245–6

Gray P (2007) Improving access to psychological therapies- the story so far. *Therapy Today*,

British Association for Counselling and Psychotherapy. **18**(2):

Horney K (1945) *Our inner conflicts*. W.W Norton, New York

Holmes J (2002) All you need is cognitive behaviour therapy? *British Medcial Journal* **324:** 288–94

Lewis JM (2000) Repairing the Bond in Important Relationships: A dynamic for Personal Maturation. *American Journal of Psychiatry* **157:** 9

Luborsky L, Crits-Christoph P (1997) *Understanding Transference: The Core Conflictual Relationship Theme Method* 2nd edn. American Psychiatric Association

Luborsky L (1984) *Principles of Psychoanalytic Psychotherapy: A Manual for Supportive-Expressive Treatment*. basic books, NY

Malan D (1963) *A Study of Brief Psychotherapy*. Tavistock, London

Malan D (1979) *Individual Psychotherapy and the Science of Psychodynamics*. Plenum, NY

Marzillier J (2004) The Myth of evidence- based psychotherapy. *The Psychologist* **17**(7):

Milewa T, Barry C (2005) Health Policy and the Politics of Evidence. *Social Policy and Administration* **39**(5): 498: 512

NICE (2004) Anxiety; management of anxiety in adults in primary, secondary and community care Clinical Guideline 22. National Institute for Clinical Excellence Publications

NICE (2004) Depression; management of depression in primary and secondary care. Clinical Guidelines 23. National Institute for Clinical Excellence Publications

NIHME (2004) *Enhanced Services Specification for Depression under the new GP contract*. NIHME

Niles B, DeAnna M, Lambert J, Wolf E (2005) Depression in Primary Care: Comorbid Disorders and Related Problems. *Journal of Clinical Psychology in Medical Settings* **12**(1): Springer Netherlands

Paxton R, Shrubb S, Griffiths H (2000) Tiered approach: matching mental health services to needs. *Journal of Mental Health* **9:** 137–44

Perry BD, Pollard RA, Blakley TL et al (1995) Childhood trauma, the neurobiology of adaptation, and 'use-dependent' development of the brain: How 'states' become 'traits'. *Infant Mental Health Journal* **16**(4): 271–91

Pietroni M (1995) The nature and aims of professional education for social workers: A postmodern perspective. In Yelloly M, Henkel M eds. *Learning and teaching in social work: Towards reflective practice*. Kingsley, London: 34–50

Perris M (2003) Psychological Therapy in Primary Care; work in progress. *Psychoanalytic Psychotherapy* **17**(1): 18–34

Proudfoot J, Ryden C, Everitt B, Shapiro D et al (2004) Clinical Efficacy of computerised cognitive-behavioural therapy for anxiety and depression in primary care: randomised control trial. *British Journal of Psychiatry* **185:** 46–54

Safran JD (1993) Breaches in the Therapeutic Alliance: An arena for negotiating authentic relatedness. *Psychotherapy* **30**(1):

Schore AN (2001) The effects of early relational trauma on right brain development, affect regulation and infant mental health. *Infant Mental Health Journal* **22**(1-2): 201–69

Slavin JH (1994) On Making Rules: Toward a Reformation of the Dynamics of Transference in Psychoanalytic Treatment. *Psychoanalytic Dialogues* **4**: 253–74

Teicher MH, Andersen SL, Polcari A et al (2003) The neurobiological consequences of early stress and childhood maltreatment. *Neuroscience & Biobehavioral Reviews* **27**(1-2): 33–44

Truax C, Mitchell K (1971) Research on certain therapist interpersonal skills in relation to process and outcome. In: Bergin A, Garfield S eds. *Handbook of Psychotherapy: an Empirical Evaluation*. Wiley, New York

Weiner B, Perry RP, Magnusson J (1988) An attributional analysis of reactions to stigmas. *Journal of Personality and Social Psychology* **55**: 738–48

Winnicot DW (1960) The theory of parent-infant relationship. In: *Maturational Processes and the Facilitating Environment*. International Universities Press, New York: 1965

CHAPTER 13

Psychosocial Interventions

Paul Rigby

Although psychotropic medication is considered to be one of the main treatment approaches for psychotic illnesses such as schizophrenia, a considerable percentage of sufferers continue to experience distressing symptoms despite taking medication, with as many as between 5% and 25% reporting that they suffer from distressing hallucinations and delusions (Jones et al, 1998). Consequently, a range of non-pharmacological treatments for people experiencing psychoses have been developed, and to some degree, evaluated.

Under the broad heading of psychosocial interventions (PSI), these adjunctive treatments to medication involve individual psychoeducational interventions, family interventions, psychological approaches to the management of symptoms such as Cognitive Behavioural Therapy and systems of service delivery such as Assertive Community Treatment (NHS Centre for Reviews and Dissemination, 2000).

What are PSI?

Rossler and Haker (2003) identify that PSI are poorly defined and that essentially interventions qualify as psychosocial if 'they are primarily directed towards a functional improvement: expanding the individual's opportunities to live in the community and to participate in societal life'.

Other definitions identify a list of key interventions 'that seek to ameliorate a user, relative or family problem associated with a psychosis using an approach based on psychological principles or addressing a change in social circumstances' (Brooker and Brabban, 2003). Brooker and Brabban (2003) go on to define PSI as 'interventions based upon a biological and psychosocial understanding of psychosis that has recovery as a goal'. The central premise of this approach is the use of a Stress Vulnerability model that proposes that psychosis is triggered and maintained by an interaction of biological, psychological and social factors. Whilst PSI definitions have been built traditionally around the strength of their evidence for clinical effectiveness, it has become accepted practice to include the following list as part of an accepted PSI package:

- The establishment of a long-term relationship with the service user and his/her family
- A comprehensive assessment of a person across the life span and life domains
- The use of structured and standardized assessment tools to inform practice
- The development of an individualized formulation to understand the person's presenting problems
- Appreciating and building upon an individual's strengths and assets
- Psychological management strategies for individuals symptoms (including Cognitive Behaviour Therapy CBT)
- Working actively with families and the social network.
- Early Intervention
- Psychopharmacology

PSI have been developed within the context of helping people who are experiencing psychosis, however the concept has now begun to be applied to other serious and enduring health problems such as dementia, chronic physical illness and palliative care. From this perspective and in this context, psychosocial care is concerned with the psychological and emotional well-being of the patient and their family/carers, including issues of self esteem, insight into and adaptation to the illness and its consequences, communication, social functioning and relationships.

The Process of Engagement and Assessment

Engagement

The processes of engagement and assessment are inextricably linked and whilst some may see the process of assessment in terms of the completion of formalized assessment tools, the overall process of assessment is a dynamic one that is inseparable from the development of a positive therapeutic relationship (Repper et al, 1994).

This process of engagement is the first step in the formation of a collaborative positive therapeutic relationship based on trust and built on hope and optimism, between a mental health professional and patient and is the vehicle by which treatment is delivered (Rapp, 1998; Repper, 2002; Gamble and Brennan, 2006).

The key features of positive therapeutic relationships have been outlined by Rapp (1998) as friendly, trusting, purposeful, reciprocal and empowering. A further influential factor to consider is the context within which the relationship develops. Environments in which the client has power and autonomy can lead to relationships which are more likely to be collaborative (Rapp, 1998; Repper, 2002).

There are a range of issues that interfere with a successful engagement process; clients may have had previous negative experiences of service provision which may include their relationships with professionals, the inflexibility of services and racial, sexual and cultural issues (Chadwick et al, 1996; Perkins and Repper, 1996; Sainsbury Centre for Mental Health, 1998). Furthermore, the nature and extent of some client's psychotic symptoms can make engagement with a mental health professionals or services problematic (Chadwick et al, 1996).

Assessment

Accurate assessment of need is essential to the planning of any intervention and whilst some may see the process of assessment in terms of the time limited completion of formalized global and specific assessment tools, the overall process is much more than this and a continuous and dynamic process (King, 2007). Through the use of a collaborative therapeutic relationship and assessment, the mental health professional aims to develop an in-depth understanding of how the illness affects the patient's life, the extent to which their ability to function is impaired and to identify what help is needed from services (Deane and Crowe, 2007; Rossler and Haker, 2003).

Whilst assessment is much more than the completion of forms, the use of a structured and systematic approach, including the use of both global and specific assessment tools, is essential to the provision of quality assessment. Through this process the aim is to clarify understanding of the presenting problems and their context, identify need and provide direction for the planning of individualised care and specific interventions (Gamble and Brennan, 2006).

There are a wide variety of structured assessment tools available that can offer practitioners guidance through the process of systematic information gathering. Such tools can be broadly divided into two categories:

- Global assessment tools that provide a broad overview of the areas being assessed
- Specific assessment tools that explore particular aspects that have been identified in the global assessment.

The use of information gathered both by the use of a structured assessment process combined with information collected as part of a developing therapeutic relationship can be used to build a 'Formulation'. A Formulation is essentially the relationship between the patient's problems, their causes and their effects (Kingdon and Turkington, 2005). The creation of a Formulation can help capture the essence of the problem by developing a shared understanding of the links between thoughts, feelings, behaviour and physiology for the patient which can help develop understanding and help provide direction for intervention (Baguley and Baguley, 2002).

Employing a Stress Vulnerability Model

The connection between exposure to stress and vulnerability to its effects are the main components of such models. Stress Vulnerability models, such as those proposed by Zubin and Spring (1977) and Strauss and Carpenter (1981), provide frameworks that can help mental health professionals and patients make sense of the way that biological, psychological and social factors may influence the onset and maintenance of serious mental illness (Brennan, 2006).

The use of stress vulnerability models can help professionals and patients normalise the experience of mental ill health in the sense that we are all exposed to differing levels of stress in our lives and at times our vulnerability to the effects of this will vary.

Stress Vulnerability models also help to explore the type and extent of the stress that an individual may be exposed to, whether their vulnerability is in born i.e. genetically determined, or acquired and the types of coping mechanisms that may be developed in response to this (Brennan, 2006; Clements and Turpin, 1992).

The Psychological Management of Symptoms

Exploring 'Delusional' Beliefs

Cognitive Behaviour Therapy (CBT) can be employed as a structured collaborative approach aimed at exploring and working with the symptoms of enduring mental ill health. The model relies upon developing a shared understanding of the relationship between thoughts, feelings and behaviours. The aim of CBT is to help the patient identify thoughts related to situations which can cause distress and to examine the evidence that supports such thoughts and explore possible alternative explanations (Everitt and Siddle, 2002).

The use of normalising rationales is an essential component of CBT approaches when working with the symptoms of psychosis. The aim of these approaches is to help to reduce the fear associated with many psychotic symptoms by examining these within the context of the extremes of human experience i.e. we can all be prone to the experience of both perceptual disturbance and thought disorder given a certain combination of circumstances (Everritt and Siddle, 2002; Kingdon and Turkington, 1991).

Through the use of CBT, the 'beliefs' which are causing distress and/or which are affecting the patient's ability to function, are explored collaboratively in a non-threatening manner (Mills, 2006). Together, the patient and 'therapist' assess the role, scope and strength of the core belief and gradually work towards exploring alternative understanding and explanations of the belief/s (Everritt and Siddle, 2002). Ultimately, the aim of any CBT is to reduce distress and disability which can result from the experience of such symptoms, but in the long term the goal is also to enhance understanding of the cognitive processes which may result in belief maintenance and to change these (Turkington and Siddle, 1998).

The evidence for the effectiveness of CBT for people with enduring mental ill health is good as there appears to be strong evidence that those patients who do receive adjunctive psychological therapy do better in terms of clinical outcomes when compared with those who do not (Tarrier et al, 1999; Sensky et al, 2000).

Working with Auditory Hallucinations (Voice Hearing)

In one of the first major reviews of treatment approaches used for auditory hallucinations, Slade and Bentall (1988) reviewed literature in relation to a total of nine 'very different and seemingly incompatible' psychological treatments, including thought stopping, reduction of sensory input and aversion therapy, which they concluded could all bring about a reduction in hallucinatory activity. Whilst suggesting that a positive expectation of change could be a single common factor in the success of all the approaches, they also identified that it was possible to group the nine treatments into three approaches; Focusing, Distraction/Counter Stimulation and Anxiety Reduction.

Focusing, as a treatment approach, involves the self monitoring of auditory hallucinations with a view to examining features such as characteristics, frequency, gender, form and attribution. Collaboratively, 'therapist' and patient explore the nature and context of the voice hearing phenomenon attempting to link the patients thoughts to their 'voices' and in the long term hopefully developing alternative explanations for the 'experience' (Bentall et al, 1994; Everritt and Siddle, 2002).

Distraction or Counter Stimulation approaches to managing voice hearing essentially involve any technique that distracts the patient away from their voice hearing experience. Such techniques may involve listening to music or speech, the use of ear plugs or activities which may provide a distraction away from the hallucinatory experience.

A number of studies have attempted to evaluate the effectiveness of a variety of distraction techniques with success being claimed for most of these in terms of the reduction of auditory hallucinations (Nelson et al, 1991; Shergill et al, 1998; Knudson and Coyle, 1999).

Anxiety Reduction

The reduction or increase of physiological arousal by the use of relaxation methods, substance use (non-prescribed drugs or alcohol) or exercise are amongst the most frequently used coping strategies that people who experience auditory hallucinations employ (Knudson and Coyle, 1999). The role of anxiety and stress as mental illness and symptom precipitators is well documented (Zubin and Spring, 1977), and the success in terms of symptom reduction for many people using anxiety reducing techniques is further evidence of the value of such approaches (Shergill et al, 1998; Knudson and Coyle, 1999) Another dimension to the benefits of anxiety reduction is provided by Haddock et al (1998) where the authors describe work which focuses upon reducing the anxiety that the auditory hallucinations induce rather than reducing the capacity of anxiety to trigger the experience.

Despite the fact that so many people with auditory hallucinations use identifiable coping strategies to reduce their impact, as many as 30% of these regard their coping strategies as ineffective (Tarrier, 1987). With this in mind, Tarrier et al (1990) describe the approach of Coping Strategy Enhancement, which aims to train people to use their existing coping strategies more effectively. A wider range of coping strategies are taught in combination with a thorough assessment and a behavioural analysis of the auditory hallucination experience which may assist sufferers to understand the origin of their voices (Yusupoff and Tarrier, 1996).

Shergill et al (1998) claim that overall there is insufficient evidence to claim that any one particular psychological intervention for auditory hallucinations is more effective than another. A range of different approaches have all demonstrated some benefit to some people with auditory hallucinations. Where such improvements have been demonstrated, evidence would suggest that this is usually related to either reducing the associated distress or increasing the individuals control of the auditory hallucinations rather than a reduction or elimination of the auditory hallucinations themselves (Shergill et al, 1998).

Working with 'Negative' Symptoms

The emphasis placed upon the so-called 'positive' symptoms of psychosis in terms of diagnosis and treatment can result in mental health professionals undervaluing and to some extent neglecting the 'negative' symptoms that effect patients (Mills et al, 2006). It is of equal importance that mental health professional's work collaboratively with patients to both prevent and alleviate negative symptoms.

Through the process of engagement and the development of a shared understanding, patients can be supported to gradually increase their activity and responsibility in an atmosphere of safety and support and work towards 'recovery' (Watkins, 1996).

As Mills et al (2006) state 'A client-centred interpersonal relationship, which focuses on the conditions of accurate empathy, non-possessive warmth and genuineness, is a prerequisite to working collaboratively with individuals to enable them to identify personal strategies for improving their motivation and confidence...'.

Promoting Concordance with Medication

The rate of non-compliance with medication regimes for people suffering from major mental illnesses such as schizophrenia has been identified as between 50-75 per cent (Gray et al, 2002). Non-adherence to prescribed medication regimes has been identified as one of the principle features of illness relapse (Meehan et al, 2007). Consequently, strategies that help to promote medication concordance may also prove to be an effective strategy of any PSI package.

There are many reasons why people may not choose to follow a prescribed medication regime and these can include; understanding of their illness, symptom level, poor relationship with mental health professionals, poor symptom control, complex medication regime, family and cultural factors as well as medication efficacy and undesirable side effects (Coffey, 1999; Harris, 2002; Gray et al, 2002).

Commonly used approaches that aim to optimise adherence include psycho-education, cognitive behavioural interventions and motivational interviewing. Psycho-educational approaches involve the education of patients and their carers about their medication, its uses, effects and side effects. However, whilst any increase in knowledge in this are amongst patients and their carers is desirable, there is no clear evidence that education alone improves adherence (Gray, 2000).

In conjunction with psycho-education, a variety of approaches have been developed called 'Compliance Therapy' which utilise a combination of components from CBT and Motivational Interviewing and which address the following issues concerning the taking of prescribed medication:

- Addressing practical issues
- Medication review
- The use of an illness timeline
- Exploring ambivalence
- Addressing common concerns about medication
- Long-term prevention (Gray et al, 2002).

Evidence to date suggests that the use of such approaches can result in improved rates of medication adherence and improved clinical outcomes (Kemp et al, 1996; Gray, 2001). However, Compliance Therapy is not without its critics who describe it as 'nothing more than surreptitious coercion' hiding behind a 'cloak of therapeutic rhetoric' (Perkins and Repper, 1998).

Working with Carers and Families

The efficacy of family work for psychosis and other serious mental illnesses is well established, with psycho educational interventions resulting in reduced relapse rates, improved medication compliance, and possible reductions in expressed emotion and social impairment (Pharoah et al, 2003).

The National Institute for Clinical Excellence (NICE) has stipulated that family work should be routinely offered to all those families 'of people with schizophrenia who are living with or who have close contact with the service user', particularly those who experience persisting symptoms (NICE, 2002), and psychoeducation and support is becoming a standard feature of other clinical guidelines in mental health (NICE, 2005; NICE, 2006).

Nurses can work with patients and their families to help increase knowledge of enduring mental ill health such as psychosis and it's effects and help families problem solve the difficulties that can arise as a result of the illness and the effects of caring.

A Structured Model of 'Family Work'

The principles of Engagement and Assessment once again provide the foundation from which collaborative 'family work' is conducted. Early meetings between 'therapists' and the family require flexibility in terms of time and venue and the adoption of a non-judgemental stance that encourages participation of all effected family members (Gamble and Brennan, 2006).

Initial meetings usually focus upon 'assessment' involving the use of both global and specific assessment tools and education which aims to address any knowledge deficits the family may have in relation to the illness and it's effects (Kuipers et al, 2002).

Once this work is completed, the structured process begins whereby areas of difficulty are worked on collectively using problem solving techniques, both in and outside of sessions, by family members using realistic, specific and mutually negotiated goals (Kuipers et al, 2002; Gamble and Brennan, 2006).

Intervening Early to Prevent Illness Relapse

It is generally accepted that intervening early in the process of psychosis brings benefits to individual patients, their carers and communities by significantly lessening the chances of relapse and chronic disability. (Birchwood et al, 1997; Falloon et al, 1998; Edwards et al, 1998). There are four elements to the approach of 'Early Intervention':

- Monitoring of those at risk
- Early detection
- Timely treatment
- Relapse prevention.

Monitoring of those at risk of developing schizophrenia would involve observing an 'at risk' group for changes in functioning or mental state. This approach is based on the evidence that prior to developing a psychotic illness people manifest 'prodromal' symptoms which can eventually evolve into a psychotic episode (Birchwood et al, 1997). As the signs of the illness begin to appear for the first time, intervention by health professionals including nurses can help all concerned manage the illness episode more effectively by offering support, education and treatment that works towards limiting the longer term effects of disability and dependency (Lloyd et al, 2007; Falloon et al, 1998).

In many cases the delay, known as the 'Duration of Untreated Psychosis' (DUP), between the onset of symptoms of psychosis and initial treatment, is between one and two years and can result in long term damage to health and reduce the chances of recovery (McGorry et al, 1999). Whilst the research is inconsistent in terms of the implications that DUP has in the long term, (Norman et al, 2005) there is general agreement that 'the bigger the time gap, the more likely patients are to have poorer outcomes across a range of measures' (NIMHE, 2003).

For people whose illness is more established, intervening early could involve collaborative work to help identify unique features of relapse, known as a 'relapse signature'. This information can be developed into a 'relapse drill' or 'protocol' which provides advice should indicators of relapse arise (Birchwood et al, 2000).

The 'Success' of PSI

The pursuit of clinical effectiveness has now become a political as well as a professional goal, and providers of healthcare are responsible for ensuring that their practice is based upon robust evidence (DH, 1998). Now part of everyday language for healthcare professionals, Clinical Effectiveness describes: 'the extent to which specific clinical interventions when deployed in the field for a particular patient or population do what they are intended to do – that is maintain and improve health and secure the greatest possible health gain from the available resources (NHS, 1996).

The concept of evidence-based practice has grown from the global desire for clinical effectiveness, in which clinicians use the best evidence available to guide their clinical decision making.

There exists a growing body of evidence for the effectiveness of PSI when dealing with many of the symptoms associated with severe mental illnesses including schizophrenia (Mueser and Bond, 2000; Cormac et al, 2003). Complementing and updating other recent reviews, Mueser and Bond (2000) conducted a review of PSI for schizophrenia focusing upon recent randomized controlled trials (RCT). They concluded that in many cases studies continued to provide support for the effectiveness of several treatment approaches and models claiming that 'these new developments in psychosocial treatment offer the promise of improving the quality of lives in persons with schizophrenia and other severe mental illnesses' (Mueser and Bond, 2000). Similarly, other major reviews supported the evidence that PSI for schizophrenia, can decrease the risk of relapse, reduce readmission rates and may even improve people's mental state (NHS Centre for Reviews and Dissemination, 2000). PSI's have received endorsement at a national policy level and are now recognized as highly desirable and effective treatment options (DH, 1999; NICE, 2002).

Similarly, other major reviews supported the evidence that PSI for schizophrenia, can decrease the risk of relapse, reduce readmission rates and may even improve people's mental state (NHS Centre for Reviews and Dissemination, 2000). However, this important area of study continues to remain under researched and well designed RCT's are needed.

However despite their proven efficacy, psychosocial interventions are not routinely integrated into clinical practice. As a result of the considerable growth in the provision of PSI training for mental health professionals, attempts have been made to evaluate their effectiveness with particular reference being made to improving the quality of care for service users. Such evaluations have identified organizational constraints as a significant impediment to the translation of training into effective clinical practice (Brooker, 2001; Brooker et al, 2003; Repper and Brooker, 2002; Smith and Velleman, 2002). These have included a lack of staff training and a variety of obstacles within service provision generally (Leff and Gamble, 1995; Fadden, 1997) such as a lack of strategic policy at a local level (Brooker, 2001), a lack of time and other resources and the unavailability of appropriate supervision (Milne et al, 2003).

The availability of appropriately skilled clinical supervision has been identified as a major barrier to the successful implementation of PSI within clinical practice (Fadden, 1997; Milne et al, 2003). As an important component of Clinical Governance, Clinical Supervision contributes to both the maintenance and improvement of patient care and is an essential tool in the professional development of all mental health professionals, providing a regular forum in which to reflect, discuss clinical practice issues and review care (Gray, 2001).

Learning Points

1. Psychosocial Interventions (PSI) are an essential adjunctive treatment to medication for a range of enduring mental health problems
2. There are four elements to the approach of 'Early Intervention': monitoring of those at risk, early detection, timely treatment; relapse prevention
3. Through the process of engagement and the use of systematic assessment methods, mental health professionals can work collaboratively with patients and their carers to provide a variety of effective interventions that can enhance clinical outcomes and improve the quality of people's lives.

References

Bagulay C, Baguley I (2002) Psychological Treatment for Anxiety and Depression in Schizophrenia. In: Harris N, Williams S, Bradshaw T, eds. *Psychosocial Interventions for People with Schizophrenia: A Practical Guide for Mental Health Workers*. Palgrave, London

Bentall R, Haddock G, Slade P (1994) Cognitive behaviour therapy for persistent auditory hallucinations: from theory to therapy. *Behaviour Therapy* **25**: 51-66

Birchwood M, McGorry P, Jackson H (1997) Early intervention in schizophrenia. *British*

Journal of Psychiatry **170**: 2-5

Birchwood M, Fowler D, Jackson C (2000) *Early Intervention in Psychosis*. John Wiley & Sons, London

Brennan G (2006) Stress vulnerability model of serious mental illness. In: Gamble C, Brennan G, eds. *Working with Serious Mental Illness: A Manual for Clinical Practice*. Elsevier, London

Brooker C (2001) A decade of evidence based training for work with people with serious mental health problems: Progress in the development of psychosocial interventions. *Journal of Mental Health* **10**(1): 17-31

Brooker C, and Brabban A (2003) Implementing Evidence Based Practice for people who experience psychosis: towards a strategic national approach. *Mental Health Review* **8**(2): 30-33

Brooker C, Saul C, Robinson J, King J, Dudley M (2003) Is training in psychosocial interventions worthwhile? Report of a psychosocial intervention trainee follow-up study. *International Journal of Nursing Studies* **40**(7): 731-747

Chadwick P, Birchwood M, Trower P (1996) *Cognitive Therapy for Delusions, Voices and Paranoia*. John Wiley, London

Clements K, Turpin N (1992) Vulnerability models and schizophrenia: the assessment and prediction of relapse. In: Birchwood M, Tarrier N, eds. *Innovations in the Psychological Management of Schizophrenia*. Wiley

Coffey M (1999) Psychosis and medication: strategies for improving adherence. *British Journal of Nursing* **8**(4): 225-230

Cormac I, Jones C, Campbell C, Silveira da Mota Neto J (2003) *Cognitive behaviour therapy for schizophrenia (Cochrane Review)*. The Cochrane Library. Issue 2, Oxford: Update Software.

Deane F, Crowe T (2007) Building and Maintaining a Recovery Focused Therapeutic Relationship. In: King R, Lloyd C, Meehan T, eds. *Handbook of Psychosocial Rehabilitation*. Blackwell, London

DH (1998) *A First Class Service: Quality in the New NHS*. DH, London

DH (1999) *Mental Health National Service Frameworks: Modern Standards and Service Models*. HMSO, London

Edwards J, Maude D, McGorry P, Harrigan S, Cocks J (1998) Prolonged recovery in first-episode psychosis. *British Journal of Psychiatry* **172**(33): 107-116

Everritt J, Siddle R (2002) Assessment and Therapeutic Interventions with Positive Psychotic Symptoms. In: Harris N, Williams S, Bradshaw T, eds. *Psychosocial Interventions for People with Schizophrenia: A Practical Guide for Mental Health Workers*. Palgrave, London

Fadden G (1998) Family intervention in psychosis. *Journal of Mental Health*. **7**(2): 115-122

Falloon I, Coverdale J, Laidlaw T, Merry S, Kydd R, Morosini P (1998) Early Intervention for Schizophrenic Disorders. *British Journal of Psychiatry* **172**(33): 107-116

Gamble C, Brennan G (2006) Working with families and informal carers. In: Gamble C, Brennan G, eds. *Working With Serious Mental Illness: A manual for clinical practice.* Elsevier, London

Gamble C, Brennan G (2006) assessments: a rationale for choosing and using. In: Gamble C, Brennan G, eds. *Working With Serious Mental Illness: A manual for clinical practice.* Elsevier, London

Gray R (2000) does patient education enhance compliance with Clozapine? A preliminary investigation. *Journal of Psychiatric and Mental Health Nursing.* **7**(3): 285-286

Gray R (2001) *A Randomised Control Trial of Medication Management training for CPN's.* Institute of Psychiatry, London

Gray R, Robson D, Bressington D (2002) Medication management for people with a diagnosis of schizophrenia. *Nursing Times* **98**(47): 38-40

Haddock G, Tarrier N, Spaulding W, Yusupoff L, Kinney C, McCarthy E (1998) Individual cognitive-behavior therapy in the treatment of hallucinations and delusions: A review. *Clinical Psychology Review* **18**(7): 821-838

Harris N (2002) Neuroleptic Drugs and their Management. In: Harris.N, Williams S, Bradshaw T, eds. P*sychosocial Interventions for People with Schizophrenia: A Practical Guide for Mental Health Workers.* Palgrave, London

Hustig H, Tran D, Hafner R, Miller R (1990) The effect of headphone music on persistent auditory hallucinations. *Behavioural Psychotherapy* **18**: 273-281

Jones C, Cormac I, Mota J, Campbell C (1998) *Cognitive behaviour therapy for schizophrenia. (Cochrane Review).* The Cochrane Library. Volume 4, Oxford

Kemp R, Hayward P, Applewhaite G, Everritt B, David A (1996) Compliance Therapy in Psychotic Patients: Randomised Control Trial. *British Medical Journal* **312**(7027): 345-349

King R (2007) Individual Assessment and the Development of a Collaborative Rehabilitation Plan. In: King R, Lloyd C, Meehan T, eds. *Handbook of Psychosocial Rehabilitation.* Blackwell, London

Kingdon D, Turkington D (1991) The use of Cognitive Behaviour Therapy with a normalizing rationale in schizophrenia. *The Journal of Nervous and Mental Disease.* **179**(4): 207-211

Kingdon D, Turkington D (2005) *Cognitive Therapy for Schizophrenia.* Guildford, London

Knudson B, Coyle A (1999) Coping strategies for hallucinations: A review. *Counselling Psychology Quarterly.* **12**(1): 25-38

Kuipers E, Leff J, Lam D (2002) *Family work for schizophrenia: A practical guide.* Gaskell, London

Leff J, Gamble C (1995) Training of Community Psychiatric Nurses in Family Work for Schizophrenia. *International Journal of Mental Health* **24**(3): 76-88

Lloyd C, King R (2007) Early Intervention, Relapse Prevention and the Promotion of Healthy Lifestyles. In: King R, Lloyd C, Meehan T, eds. *Handbook of Psychosocial Rehabilitation*. Blackwell, London

McGorry P, Jackson H (1999) *The Recognition and Management of Early Psychosis: A Preventative Approach*. Cambridge University Press, Canbridge

Meehan T, McCombes S, Stedman T (2007) Integrating Psychosocial Rehabilitation and Pharmacology. In: King R, Lloyd C, Meehan T, eds, *Handbook of Psychosocial Rehabilitation*. Blackwell, London

Mills J (2006) Dealing with Voices and Strange Thoughts. In: Gamble C, Brennan G, eds. *Working With Serious Mental Illness: A manual for clinical practice*. Elsevier, London

Mills J, Kerr S, Goldspink S (2006) Dealing with blankness and deadness. In: Gamble C, Brennan G, eds. *Working With Serious Mental Illness: A manual for clinical practice*. Elsevier, London

Milne D, Carpenter J, Lombardo C, Dickinson C (2003) *Psychosocial Interventions: External evaluation of programme at Sunderland University*. Northern Centre for Mental Health

Mueser K, Bond G (2000) Psychosocial treatment approaches for schizophrenia. *Current Opinion in Psychiatry* **13**(1): 27-35

NHS (1996) *Promoting Clinical Effectiveness: A Framework for Action in and Throughout the NHS*. Department of Health, London.

NICE (2002) S*chizophrenia: Core interventions in the treatment and management of schizophrenia in primary and secondary care. Clinical Guideline 1*. NICE, London

NICE (2005) *Obsessive Compulsive Disorder. Clinical Guideline 31*. NICE, London

NICE (2006) *Biploar Disorder: The management of bipolar disorder in adults, children and adolescents in primary and secondary care Clinical Guideline 38*. NICE, London

Nelson H, Thrasher S, Barnes T (1991) Practical ways of alleviating auditory hallucinations. *British Medical Journal* **302**: 327

NHS Centre for Reviews and Dissemination (2000) Psychosocial interventions for schizophrenia. *Effective Health Care* **6**(3): 1-8

NIMHE (2003) *Early Intervention for People with Psychosis*. NIMHE

Norman R, Lewis S, Marshall M (2005) Duration of untreated psychosis and its relationship to clinical outcome. *British Journal of Psychiatry* **187**(48): 19-23

Perkins R, Repper J (1996) *Working Alongside People with Long Term Mental Health Problems*. Stanley Thornes

Perkins R, Repper J (1998) Softly, softly. *Mental Health Care* **2**(2): 70

Pharoah F, Mari J, Streiner D (2003) *Family intervention for schizophrenia (Cochrane Review)*. The Cochrane Review. Issue 2, Oxford; Updated Software.

Rapp C (1998) The Strengths Model: Case Management with People Suffering from Severe and Persistent Mental Illness. In: Rapp C, ed. *Engagement and Relationship: A New Partnership*. Oxford University Press, Oxford

Repper J, Ford R, Cooke A (1994) How can nurses build trusting relationships with people who have severe and long term mental health problems? Experiences of case managers and their clients. *Journal of Advanced Nursing* :1096-1104

Repper J (2002) The Helping Relationship. In: Harris N, Williams S, Bradshaw T, eds. *Psychosocial Interventions for People with Schizophrenia: A Practical Guide for Mental Health Workers*. Palgrave, London

Repper D, Brooker C (2002) *Avoiding the Wash Out: Developing the organizational context to increase the uptake of evidence based practice for psychosis*. Northern Centre for Mental Health

Rossler W, Haker H (2003) Conceptualizing psychosocial interventions. *Current Opinion in Psychiatry* **16**: 709-712

Sensky T, Turkington D, Kingdon D, Scott J, Scott J, Siddle R, O'Carroll M, Barnes T (2000) A randomized controlled trial of cognitive-behavioural therapy for persistent symptoms in schizophrenia resistant to medication. *Archives of General Psychiatry* **57**(92): 165-172

Shergill S, Murrary R, McGuire P (1998) Auditory Hallucinations: a review of psychological treatments. *Schizophrenia Research* **32**: 137–150

Slade P, Bentall R (1988) *Sensory Deception: A Scientific Analysis of Hallucinations*. Croom Helm

Smith G, Velleman R (2002) Maintaining a Family Work for Psychosis service by recognizing the barriers to implementation. *Journal of Mental Health* **11**(5): 471-479

Tarrier N (1987) An investigation of residual psychotic symptoms in discharged schizophrenic patients. *British Journal of Clinical Psychology*. **26**: 141-143

Tarrier N, Harwood S, Yusupoff L, Beckett R, Baker A (1990) Coping Strategy Enhancement (CSE): A method of treating residual schizophrenic symptoms. *Behavioural Psychotherapy* **18**: 283-293

Tarrier N, Wittkowski A, Kinney C, McCarthy E, Morris J, Humphreys L (1999) Durability of the effects of cognitive-behavioural therapy in the treatment of chronic schizophrenia: 12-month follow-up. *British Journal of Psychiatry* **174**: 500-504

The Sainsbury Centre for Mental Health (1998) *Keys to Engagement; Review of care for people who are hard to engage with services*. Sainsbury Centre for Mental Health

Turkington D, Siddle R (1998) Cognitive Therapy for the Treatment of Delusions. *Advances in Psychiatric Treatment* **4**: 235-242

Watkins J (1996) *Living with Schizophrenia: A holistic approach to understanding, preventing and recovering from negative symptoms*. Hill of Content.

Yusupoff L, Tarrier N (1996) Coping Strategy Enhancement for Persistent Hallucinations and Delusions. In: Haddock G, Slade P, eds. *Cognitive-Behavioural Interventions with*

Psychotic Disorders. Routledge, London

Zubin J, Spring B (1977) Vulnerability — a New View of Schizophrenia. *Journal of Abnormal Psychology* **86**(2): 260-266

CHAPTER 14

Models of Nursing

James Dooher and Oduth Chooramun

Nursing models are out of fashion, and the changing context of rehabilitative care has seen a decline in the interest, understanding and application of nursing models. Aggleton and Chalmers (2000) noted that the role of the nurse practitioner has 'changed', however it seems that the added value a nursing model brings to the process of care delivery has been lost within the change process. Tomey and Allgood (2002) suggested that the evolution of nursing theories has been a search for nursing substance, and this reluctance to consider nursing models reflects a loss of substance to the range of care delivery options which should be availed to clients in the rehabilitation process.

The impact of this change is most evident in the psychiatric rehabilitative nursing settings. Mental health practitioners in these settings have an important role to play in the light of the current modernisation plan of the NHS mental health services, which now seem to be a key government initiative.

It is generally asserted that the nurse practitioner has a 'unique place within rehabilitation team' (Williams, 1993). Hence, for the mental health nurse working in the rehabilitative nursing settings, this amounts to the enduring task of promoting independence and restoring the functions of the enduring mentally ill clients to the pre-illness level as close as possible to an optimum level. Empowering clients to rediscover, or perhaps reach for the first time, their optimum functioning level, is a challenge that demands personalised needs assessment as a prerequisite. Nursing models may really help this process but are considered by many to restrict creativity and inhibit the art of nursing itself. McKenna (1997) suggested that theories should not be accepted unquestioningly, and that any analysis of their usefulness may be difficult as most nursing theories are abstract.

The rehabilitation and resettlement of clients with enduring mental health problems has never been a straightforward matter, and it has posed a challenge to service providers, particularly in a climate of social political and economic reforms which are often contradictory.

The Victorian penchant for fresh air and an isolationist approach to mental illness saw the development of large institutions, mainly placed outside the major centres of population, and it was not until the White Paper *Working for Patients and Caring for People* (DH, 1988) that alternatives were actively considered.

The subsequent de-centralisation and closure of these institutions has seen a completely new vista in the way treatment resources are being targeted to these clients. Consequently, it could be argued that the role and scope of practice within the rehabilitative nursing practice has changed significantly, with implications for all concerned. This has meant that a greater emphasis is being placed on more community-oriented aspects of care, rather than hospital-based services. One can of course argue that despite all these changes the need for people with mental health problem to be admitted for psychiatric in-patient care for acute treatment of relapse, or initial mental health breakdown, will continue to generate the demand for hospital based care. For this reason, it could be argued that habilitation and rehabilitation will always be in demand, and that professionals working within this arena have an enormous task and contribution to make.

Community Model

The option of long-term continuing care is increasingly under pressure (except for those with a severe and enduring mental health problem), and options of community-based living, be it wholly independent or supervised is, an increasing reality. The assessment of needs and subsequent care delivery should take place within a systematic, planned and organised manner that demonstrates application of research findings that underpin the care delivery. It is thus imperative that this care package is delivered within the framework of a multidisciplinary approach in which the mental health nurses playing a key role in its implementation and direction.

The use of an appropriate nursing model of care and the subsequent evaluation of the appropriateness of the model of care used is a highly desirable prerequisite for the delivery of quality care, tailored to meet the need of clients with an enduring mental health problem. It is argued that a model of care can assist in ascertaining the kind of intervention 'best suited to the needs of the clients' and can thus 'contribute to the decision of who should intervene, and in what way' (Aggleton and Chalmers, 2000).

Models also promote independence which can, on occasions, mean professionals taking risks in allowing a vulnerable adult to pursue the lifestyle they choose, thereby offering them independence within the constraints of their incapacity and, importantly, maintains them in their own home or community. Some risk taking must be seen as essential if the caring agencies are to avoid shutting a vulnerable person away from the challenges and opportunities of 'normal' life in an attempt to protect them.

During local care plan audits and profiles to ascertain the areas suitability for student placement, models have often not been applied in practice because of unnecessary jargon and overcomplicated terminology, which leads to confusion and misinterpretation. On the other hand literal interpretation and an almost spiteful adherence to the framework of a model can ensure its unsuitability. The sabotage may stem from a conflict between the ideology of the model and the nurses own professional and ethical standpoint. It may well be the ubiquitous paperwork versus patient care debate, or it could be that the nurses are simply bored by prescriptive instruction and reject model as a means of gaining control of their own professional space.

Introducing a Model to Care

Conversely, certain practice areas are receptive to the idea of applying nursing models in the delivery of care to clients. Certain models, such as for example Roy's Adaptation and Orem's (1980) Model for Self Care, are being used quite usefully. However it is worth noting that some degree of inconsistencies and ambiguities exist in this domain.

As link lecturers we work with the clinical placement areas to offer support to students during their clinical allocation. The students are required to submit a written care study based on the framework of the nursing process using an appropriate model of care — quite frequently in the line of pursuance of students' enquiries and concerns with the respective supervisors in relation to the students' assessed work. In our experience we have the impression that some clinical practitioners are either not well versed with the philosophy of care model, or in some cases they are not receptive to the idea of using a model of care in their practice settings, without being able to offer any valid and justifiable support for their reservation. The common argument being that '*we have tried it before*'.

The benefits of introducing a model are often outweighed by the difficulties. These difficulties are often intangible: for example the nurse's capacity to find — and then understand — a suitable model; and his/her ability to interpret the model.

Gaining the support and concordance of the client is a vital yet often overlooked block to successful implementation. Nursing consistency and continuity of care plan delivery and support from the multidisciplinary team are essential building blocks for care. Without these essential elements even the most basic care plan will be difficult to implement.

One thing that is fairly clear is that models of care have been in existence in clinical practice for many years. Their utilisation or resistance to apply them has remained a matter for the multidisciplinary team to debate and decide. One can only argue that the choice of a model does not necessarily have to be a rigid one. A model suited to the needs of the respective clients and the mental health nurse being receptive, comfortable and conversant with the appropriateness of its philosophy and application, is a sufficiently good criterion for the selection of a model for the practice setting. It could however be said that the nurse practitioner in this situation may be faced with equally attractive alternatives. It is argued that 'choosing between models is something one does intuitively as an act of personal preferences' which in reality may not always solve all the day-to-day problems of the clients, the nurse and the practice setting (Aggleton and Chalmers, 2000).

What then could be the alternative? The alternative to choosing from models already in existence may well lie in the nurse practitioners' critical thinking abilities, resolute conviction and professional aspirations. A demonstration of commitment to the degree of innovation and creativity in designing and producing their own version of a model of care that could be put together with active participation and contribution of the various inter-professional discipline should be seen as an attractive proposition.

Hogson and Simpson (1999) suggest that the 'basic starting point for a model is a statement of the beliefs and values that underpin it'. Thus within the rehabilitation setting the starting point may well be a critical appraisal and analysis of the areas, which is a framework of care that embodies the philosophical beliefs and values upon which nursing care is delivered. This should encompass the therapeutic milieu of the respective setting.

Hence a range of models could be scrutinised and ideas can be put together to produce the format of a specific model of care best suited to the needs of the clients, the practice setting, the inter-professional discipline and management. The fact that it has the model would have been conceived with the contribution of the inter-professional team and the involvement of the managers, it would have the benefits of being adapted to fit the given situation. It could be said that in order for this initiative to materialise and the outcome become positive, the attitude of the staff, team leaders, and managers must at the very least be moderately positive towards theory-based nursing. Receptiveness to an application of nursing theories or models to guide practice may be greatly influenced by those deemed 'in charge' and their expert knowledge and experience are paramount to the success. Fawcett (1995) observes that:

> '...the discipline of nursing can survive and advance only if nurses celebrate their own heritage by adopting explicit conceptual models of nursing and nursing theories to guide their activities'.
>
> *Fawcett, 1995*

It could be argued that an initiative of this magnitude has the added advantage of bringing harmony and cohesiveness within the team. This could lead to the eventual emergence of a solid and dynamic team spirit. Hence the work of the team will be enriched and a greater degree of job satisfaction and a high standard of morale will prevail, as the credibility and professional status of the team will be greatly enhanced.

Moreover, a good communication network that will facilitate an effective feedback loop and consistency will be established. This will inevitably lead to the development and maintenance of good record-keeping and an overall improved level of quality documentation. This will no doubt enhance not only the image, but also the robustness, of auditing outcomes. All these can be used as a valid measure of care delivered. Hence the nature of theoretical thinking and the intellectual and cognitive actions of the team will be highlighted in a very positive perspective.

Why Would a Nursing Model be Useful?

Nursing models by their very nature focus upon a specific theme or problem within an area of practice, and it is this very focus which undermines any universal applicability. This in turn opens up any model to criticism of being too restrictive and in direct conflict with individualised client patient care. Models exist to protect the practitioner from the vagaries of intuition, stereotypical practice or inconsistent delivery of care. They introduce a scientific element to nursing interventions.

However, can models of nursing such as the Neuman Model (1972), the Systems Model, the Roy Adaptation Model (1976) or Orem Self Care Model (1971) be helpful to nurses? Do they act as a guideline to inform intervention and care, or do they hamper a nurse's development of an individual style, inhibit professional growth and stifle creativity?

It was not until the mid 1970s that the meta-paradigms of nursing began to be interpreted as models, A range of authors (Johnson, 1974; Reihl and Roy, 1974,1980; Reilly, 1974) attempted to make sense of some of the grand theories that had been debated since the work of Florence Nightingale (1859).

It could be said that the real benefit of the array of available models are in that they have assisted to advance notions, ideas and debate about the nature of nursing. Models identify some of the qualitatively different ways nursing can be expressed and their usefulness in affirming the possibility for a depth of philosophical and conceptual explanation within the various domain of nursing, However, all this is useless if these ideas are not translated onto practice. A model should be an abstraction of reality which provides a way to visualise reality in order to simplify thinking. Perhaps the perceived complexity of grand theories or meta-paradigms has put people off, yet as Fawcett (1995) observes, most models adopt simple elements such as 'nursing or caring', 'health', 'person' and 'environment', and dividing a care plan under these domains is clearly both simple and useful. Fawcett (1989) proposed that:

'...the utility of conceptual models comes from the organisation they provide for thinking for, observations and for interpreting what is seen; providing a systematic structure and a rationale for activities'.

Fawcett, 1989

However, the current trend to provide care outside of these parameters is testimony to the failure of the nursing model to positively influence practice.

Learning Points

1. The rehabilitation and resettlement of clients with enduring mental health problems has never been a straightforward matter, and it has posed a challenge to service providers, particularly in a climate of social political and economic reforms which are often contradictory
2. The use of an appropriate nursing model of care and the subsequent evaluation of the appropriateness of the model of care used is a highly desirable prerequisite for the delivery of quality care
3. Models promote independence
4. A range of models could be scrutinised and ideas can be put together to produce the format of a specific model of care best suited to the needs of the clients, the practice setting, the inter-professional discipline and management.

References

Fawcett J (1989) *Analysis and Evaluation of Conceptual Models*. FA Davies, Philadelphia

Fawcett (1995) *Analysis and Evaluation of Theories of Nursing*. FA Davies, Philadelphia

Orem DE (1971) *Concepts of Practice*. McGraw Hill, New York

Reilly DE (1975) Why a conceptual Framework? *Nursing Outlook* **23**: 566–9

Riehl JP, Roy C (1974) *Conceptual models for nursing practice*. Appleton-Centaury-Crofts, New York

Riehl JP, Roy C (1980) *Conceptual models for nursing practice*. 2nd edn. Appleton-Centaury-Crofts, New York

Roy C (1976) *Introduction to Nursing: An adaption model*. Prentice-Hall, Englewood Cliffs, New Jersey

McKenna H (1997) *Nursing Theories and Models*. Routledge, London: 222

Neuman B, Young RJ (1972) A model for teaching total person aproach to patient problems. *Nursing Research* **21:** 264–9

Nightingale F (1859) *Notes on Nursing: What it is and what it is not*. London Harrison. Reprint, 1948. Lippincot, Philadelphia

Tomey AM, Allgood MR (2002) *Nursing Theorists and Their Work*. Mosby, Missouri

Wiedenbach E (1964) *Clinical nursing: A helping art*. Springer, New York

CHAPTER 15

Conclusion

James Dooher

Like physical health, mental health is something we all have, and good mental health is something that we all strive for. All too often, a person may only consider their mental health when things go wrong.

When our mental health is challenged, it does not necessarily mean we are mentally ill; an episode of poor mental health can just be a one-off event in a similar way to backache, tennis elbow or a twisted ankle. With the right treatment can be effectively resolved.

Mental health nurses are in the frontline in providing support to people with mental health problems, working with the multidisciplinary team to coordinate and provide care. The central core of mental health nursing skills is the ability to form one-to one personal 'therapeutic' relationships with people. This, coupled with the nurses ability to communicate and utilise their own personality within a caring, supportive and professional relationship, is the basis of this branch of nursing. These qualities are framed in the context of the workplace which requires imaginative deployment staff and resources, good leadership, fair pay and career development to make a key contribution to the changes required of future mental health services.

Overall, we need to develop capable mental health nurses who are able to deliver services that effectively meet the needs of the people who use them.

Mental health workers from many different disciplines recognise that they share knowledge, skills and values that cross health and social care.

The Ten Essential Shared Capabilities for Mental Health Practice

Working in Partnership

Developing and maintaining constructive working relationships with service users, carers, families, colleagues, lay people and wider community networks. Working positively with any tensions created by conflicts of interest or aspiration that may arise between the partners in care.

Respecting Diversity

Working in partnership with service users, carers, families and colleagues to provide care and interventions that not only make a positive difference but also do so in ways that respect and value diversity including age, race, culture, disability, gender, spirituality and sexuality.

Practising Ethically

Recognising the rights and aspirations of service users and their families, acknowledging power differentials and minimising them whenever possible. Providing treatment and care that is accountable to service users and carers within the boundaries prescribed by national (professional), legal and local codes of ethical practice.

Challenging Inequality

Addressing the causes and consequences of stigma, discrimination, social inequality and exclusion on service users, carers and mental health services. Creating, developing or maintaining valued social roles for people in the communities they come from.

Promoting Recovery

Working in partnership to provide care and treatment that enables service users and carers to tackle mental health problems with hope and optimism and to work towards a valued lifestyle within and beyond the limits of any mental health problem.

Identifying People's Needs and Strengths

Working in partnership to gather information to agree health and social care needs in the context of the preferred lifestyle and aspirations of service users their families, carers and friends.

Providing Service User Centred Care

Negotiating achievable and meaningful goals; primarily from the perspective of service users and their families. Influencing and seeking the means to achieve these goals and clarifying the responsibilities of the people who will provide any help that is needed, including systematically evaluating outcomes and achievements.

Making a Difference

Facilitating access to and delivering the best quality, evidence-based, values-based health and social care interventions to meet the needs and aspirations of service users and their families and carers.

Promoting Safety and Positive Risk Taking

Empowering the person to decide the level of risk they are prepared to take with their health and safety. This includes working with the tension between promoting safety and positive risk taking, including assessing and dealing with possible risks for service users, carers, family members, and the wider public.

Personal Development and Learning

Keeping up-to-date with changes in practice and participating in life-long learning, personal and professional development for one's self and colleagues through supervision, appraisal and reflective practice.

The Themes in this book echo the aspirations set out in the *Ten Essential Shared Capabilities for Mental Health Practice* (DH, 2004), and attempt to support the worthy aspirations contained within it. We have paid particular attention to the therapeutic relationship and its manifestation in a variety of contexts, placing the patient at the centre of all activity. We have hopefully provided the reader with a balanced accessible series of views, not overly burdened with heavy analytical theory.

References

DH (2004) *Ten Essential Shared Capabilities*. Department of Health, London

Index